Qualitative Metasynthesis

T0352796

Qualitative Metasynthesis presents a research method developed for upcycling and synthesis of qualitative primary studies, aimed at researchers within medicine and health sciences.

This book demonstrates why and how qualitative metasynthesis can be a method for reuse and expansion of medical knowledge. It presents the principles of metasynthesis as a qualitative research method, so that the reader can assess whether this is a research strategy that fits the aim of their study. The author offers practical advice for conducting research using this methodology. The presentation is illustrated by a study carried out by the author and collaborators, reflecting on real-life challenges and solutions as an example of meta-ethnography, one of the most frequently used strategies for qualitative metasynthesis. The author also refers to systematic reviews, a methodology developed within in the tradition of evidence-based medicine, discussing strengths, weaknesses and pitfalls of this methodology. Rooted in the interpretative paradigm, qualitative metasynthesis challenges several of the principles from the evidence-based medicine tradition, offering reflections on challenges when epistemologically very different methodologies intersect.

This book should be considered essential reading for anyone carrying out qualitative research within the fields of medicine, health and social care.

Kirsti Malterud, MD PhD, was a general practitioner for 35 years, combined with academic work as a researcher at Uni Research/NORCE Research Centre and a Professor of General Practice at the University of Bergen, Norway. Her list of research publications is extensive, with empirical studies about vulnerable groups of patients as well as methodological contributions on qualitative research methods.

Qualitative Metasynthesis
A Research Method for Medicine and Health Sciences

Kirsti Malterud

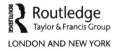

Routledge
Taylor & Francis Group

LONDON AND NEW YORK

First published in English 2019
by Routledge
4 Park Square, Milton Park, Abingdon, Oxon OX14 4RN
605 Third Avenue, New York, NY 10017

First issued in paperback 2023

Routledge is an imprint of the Taylor & Francis Group, an informa business

© 2019 Kirsti Malterud

Translated from Norwegian into English by Kirsti Malterud
The right of Kirsti Malterud to be identified as author of this
work has been asserted by her in accordance with sections
77 and 78 of the Copyright, Designs and Patents Act 1988.

Published in Norwegian by Universitetsforlaget 2017

Publisher's Note
The publisher has gone to great lengths to ensure the quality of this
reprint but points out that some imperfections in the original copies
may be apparent.

British Library Cataloguing-in-Publication Data
A catalogue record for this book is available from the British Library

Library of Congress Cataloging-in-Publication Data
A catalog record has been requested for this book

ISBN-13: 978-0-367-13418-1 (hbk)
ISBN-13: 978-1-03-265354-9 (pbk)
ISBN-13: 978-0-429-02634-8 (ebk)

DOI: 10.4324/9780429026348

Typeset in Times New Roman
by codeMantra

Contents

Abbreviations

Abbreviation	Full concept	Explanation
CASP	Critical Appraisal Skills Programme	Checklist for qualitative studies
CERQual	Confidence in the evidence from reviews of qualitative research	Method for grading evidence quality and strength of recommendations in qualitative metasyntheses
CFS/ME	Chronic fatigue syndrome/Myalgic encephalopathy	
CINAHL	The Cumulative Index to Nursing and Allied Health Literature	Database of research literature
CMO	Context (C), mechanism (M), outcome (O)	Analysis with realist synthesis focusing on conditions for intervention
COREQ	Consolidated criteria for reporting qualitative research	Checklist for qualitative studies
EBM	Evidence-based medicine	
ENTREQ	Enhancing Transparency in Reporting the Synthesis of Qualitative Research	Checklist for reporting qualitative metasyntheses
EQUATOR	Enhancing the quality and transparency of health research	Flow sheet for reporting literature searches and reviews
GRADE	Grading of recommendations assessment, development and evaluation	Method for grading evidence quality and strength of recommendations in systematic reviews
GT	Grounded theory	A method for qualitative analysis

(Continued)

Abbreviation	*Full concept*	*Explanation*
MEDLINE	Medical literature analysis and retrieval system online	Database of research literature
MM	Mixed methods	
NHD	Nursing home doctor	
NOKC	Norwegian Knowledge Centre for the Health Services	Independent government unit
PICO	Population-Intervention-Comparison-Outcome	Acronym developed for literature searches of systematic reviews of intervention studies
PROSPERO	International prospective register of systematic reviews	Database of systematic reviews
QMARS	Qualitative Meta-analysis Article Reporting Standards	Reporting standards developed by American Psychological Association
QUADAS	Quality Assessment of Diagnostic Accuracy Studies	Methodology for systematic reviews of studies of diagnostic tests
RCT	Randomized Controlled Trial	
SPIDER	Sample, Phenomenon of Interest, Design, Evaluation, Research type	Acronym developed for literature searches for qualitative metasyntheses
SR	Systematic review	

Preface

After some decades of engagement with qualitative research methods in medicine and health sciences, I have become increasingly preoccupied by knowledge as something that is built by communities of researchers. With previous knowledge as our points of departure, we want to challenge the old knowledge and develop new. Too often, though, we start nearly from scratch, as if we were the first ever to explore a certain problem. To obtain an overview of the research literature is an important precondition to find out what is missing to set out on one's own project. Summing up what we come across in a systematic way may also evolve into an independent research project. Qualitative metasynthesis is a specific research method for the systematic review, upcycling and synthesis of qualitative primary studies.

With this book, I am addressing researchers from medicine and health sciences, especially PhD students and postdocs with background knowledge from qualitative studies. The methodological traditions in these disciplines are heavily influenced by biomedicine, epidemiology and quantitative research. Special attention to the presentation of and arguments for the interpretative paradigm underlying qualitative methods is still needed. Evidence-based medicine has had a particularly powerful impact on the methodology of systematic reviews within this field, especially regarding literature search and selection and ideas of standardization and generalization, originally developed for very different kinds of data and analysis. Important paradigmatic challenges are raised by this situation and deserve the specific discussion offered in this book. Still, the book is not about systematic reviews in general – they are discussed only as far as their methodology frames qualitative metasynthesis.

The book is intended to contribute to the elaboration of qualitative methodology skills, to demonstrate the use of qualitative metasynthesis as a tool for upcycling and expanding the medical field of knowledge and to offer practical advice for conducting these kinds of studies. I present principles and procedures specific to metasynthesis as a qualitative method, giving the reader an opportunity to consider whether it is a research strategy that is suited to the research aim of a given study.

This book refers to my selection of empirical studies as well as texts about methodological and theoretical issues which are reflected in a comprehensive list of references. My aim is to present principles and procedures for the most frequently used methods in the context of other available strategies. I selected Noblit and Hare's meta-ethnography as the method to be presented in more detail, but I am not offering a comprehensive overview of all existing strategies for qualitative metasynthesis.

My writing process has itself been a kind of qualitative meta-metasynthesis, in which I have tried to translate the different contributions into one another in order to develop new connections. I have emphasized the presentation of practical procedures and issues related to sustainability of knowledge with qualitative metasynthesis as a tool. Furthermore, I have taken the opportunity to reflect on and discuss the scientific strengths, weaknesses and pitfalls related to these strategies. A study in which I participated serves as an example throughout the book to elucidate specific challenges and solutions.

However, this book is not only meant to be a practical textbook. Qualitative metasynthesis challenges several of the paradigms in which the evidence-based medicine tradition and the systematic review methodology are entrenched. Such considerations offer a point of departure for reflections on the most urgent challenges arising when two epistemologically very different methodologies intersect.

I am grateful to many people for their support, advice and specific contributions. My workplace, the Research Unit for General Practice/NORCE Norwegian Research Centre, Bergen, Norway directed by Sabine Ruths, offers daily recognition and encouragement. Anette Fosse, a general practitioner in Mo i Rana, Norway, opened the door to her own PhD project about the role of the nursing home doctor at the end of life and agreed to have her project serve as an example in the book. Signe Flottorp and Lillebeth Larun from the Norwegian Institute of Public Health have provided valuable comments along the way. Randi Bolstad and Regina Küfner Lein at the University of Bergen Library, Department of Medicine and Dentistry, have shared their professional skills as research librarians. Countless discussions in the cross-disciplinary "Knowledge, power and health services" research group with the always optimistic Anne Karen Bjelland and Kari Tove

Elvbakken raised many important questions. Sally Thorne and Trish Greenhalgh encouraged the translation from Norwegian to English and commented on ethical regulations and approvals.

Fortunately, my supporters do not agree about everything, and as the author, I take full responsibility for the text and its content. Berlin, Germany, was a wonderful place to find a deeper understanding, concentration, inspiration and joy first in writing the book in its original Norwegian version and in finishing the translation to English two years later.

Finally, I wish to thank many researchers I have not met – the authors of the research articles I used as the foundation for writing this book. Building stone by stone, we may together contribute to progress and development instead of standing still or walking in circles.

Bergen, May 2019
Kirsti Malterud

1 Utilization and upcycling of existing research knowledge

We do not have to start from scratch

Research should build on the existing base of knowledge. As researchers we acquaint ourselves with, challenge and extend the understanding and insights mediated by those who have come before us. A thorough and critical literature review can constitute a point of departure for new projects and serve as the basis for independent and innovative research that upcycles existing knowledge by finding new uses for and value in that knowledge. Synopses and syntheses of existing research knowledge can also offer new insights beyond what we already know, for what we already know is what we generally notice in the evidence we encounter. Systematic reflection is therefore an important precondition for upcycling existing research knowledge to fulfil scientific criteria.

Qualitative studies – an open mind, but no blank slates

Qualitative research methods are often used to explore themes with limited research evidence. We draw conclusions by moving from the particular to the general, focusing on subjectivity during data collection and *interpretation* and analysis (Malterud, 2001b, 2017b). The field of *epistemology* focuses on knowledge about knowledge. The epistemological preconditions for qualitative research methods are rooted in the *interpretative paradigm* (see Chapter 4), but our interpretations are not arbitrary. They must be reached with professional reflexivity in order to become research knowledge (Alvesson & Sköldberg, 2009).

Qualitative methods are better suited to developing new questions than to repeating previous answers. As the explicit aim is to develop original and relevant knowledge, the qualitative researcher often takes up the position of explorer or traveller (Kvale, 1996), with a feeling of entering a jungle in which nobody has previously tread. This researcher identity is supported by using *inductive* approaches with qualitative research methods. Being researchers, however, we do not have blank slates when we enter the field and encounter empirical data.

To be sure, some qualitative methodology traditions argue that the best point of departure is to start the research project with an open mind and enter the field without any preconceptions. I disagree with this position. We certainly do not start with answers decided on in advance, but it is not possible to wipe the slate entirely clean and reset human imagination and experience (Morse, 1994). As human beings, we always take along inner images of how the world looks as to the questions we want to answer or elucidate. We always belong to some context or other of existing knowledge and understanding. The qualitative researcher might therefore need an extra reminder that we do not need to start from scratch every time we set off on a new research project.

Research waste or exploiting knowledge capital?

The concept of *research waste* has appeared on the academic agenda in recent years (Chalmers et al., 2014). We are wasting research if we do not sensibly use what is already there. Knowledge is power and should be shared. Within the academic community, research evidence is regarded as a joint asset, and we can contribute to the further development of knowledge capital by the best possible utilization of knowledge provided by other researchers. Instead of starting from scratch, we should therefore establish an overview of existing evidence, taking a qualified and critical perspective (Britten et al., 2017). Independent of a research aim or method, the project will benefit from a comprehensive literature search as a point of departure to identify the foundation and establish an appropriate starting point.

In this way, I can first pay due respect to my colleagues and prevent arrogance. Otherwise, my enthusiastic starting mood might seduce me into thinking that I am the first or the only or the best researcher to explore the topic in question. A reality orientation can support a calming, sobering counterbalance when I find my own research question to be amazingly original, and I will often discover that somebody already has been close to the issue I want to explore. Perhaps an excellent study has recently been published, illuminating my aim better than I could. Instead of seeing this as having lost a competition, I can rather imagine that I am participating in a relay race in which I recognize the teammate who passes me the baton as a great point of departure for my own leg.

Second, I am spared much unnecessary extra work by finding out what research has already been done about the issue. When I can stand on the shoulders of others, I do not have to start from zero myself (Moher et al., 2016). By means of a comprehensive literature search, it is likely that I will meet hitherto unknown like-minded colleagues – researchers from different parts of the world who share my interest and have already explored parts of the topic that are perhaps not exactly what I want to pursue myself. Hence, I can obtain good raw materials that help me to mould my research aim without simply repeating what is already known. I can also use my recently acquired insights to make connections for further collaboration. In this way, the potential for developing more original knowledge is enhanced, which will provide a bonus from the editors and reviewers who will assess the contributions as to readability and originality.

Third, a literature review can always give access to learning and new insights, even in a subject that I think I already know well. New publications may appear, presenting questions, perspectives, methods or results that push me forward with new ideas about my field of research or my plans. Such inspirations are more easily put into practice when they appear early in the research process. Closer to the end, more is needed to substantially change my mind or direction.

Recycling, upcycling and sustainable management of knowledge resources

Recycling, a concept developed and promoted by the environmental movement, means that items that have apparently become redundant or unnecessary are used again instead of simply being thrown away (Rosvold, 2012). Recycling is a logical response to waste and a measure to counteract the preventable destruction of valuable commodities and environmental contamination. Two students furnish their home with a couch and a dining table set aside by a middle-aged couple. Dresses from the 1980s become popular retro clothing among hipsters in 2018. Useful objects are being utilized in a new context, and instead of becoming garbage or contamination, old items are given new opportunities in new frames. *Upcycling* means "to upcycle (something) in such a way that the resulting product is of a higher value than the original item" (Merriam Webster Dictionary). This is something other than the transformation of garbage, where objects are dissolved into raw materials and reused in something completely different, as when soda bottles become a fleece sweater.

The idea of upcycling may also be applied to knowledge. Today, vast amounts of research evidence are produced that deserve upcycling instead of being laid aside or ignored. As researchers, we have a responsibility to ensure the best possible exploitation of the resources we control, be it research funding or knowledge capital. The environmental researcher and philosopher Robert Frodeman suggests that, in an era characterized by overproduction of knowledge which is insufficiently utilized (Frodeman, 2014), we should assess the development of knowledge as we do with environmental problems. He writes about sustainable knowledge as an essential precondition for crossdisciplinarity. With Frodeman's notion in mind, we can regard knowledge as a renewable resource.

In this book, I will use such ideas as arguments for the sustainable upcycling of research evidence. I am not proposing a transformation of the original product into something totally different and unrecognizable. We are dealing with methods for the development of knowledge where research evidence is valued as a resource in such a way that the core of the knowledge is elaborated but still preserved. Qualitative metasynthesis – the subject of this book – is one of the several possible strategies to achieve this purpose (Malterud, 2017a).

Sustainable development is defined as development in which "harvesting or using a resource so that the resource is not depleted or permanently damaged" (Merriam Webster Dictionary). *Sustainability* implies accountability for the future through the responsible use of current resources. The concept of sustainability includes both overarching strategies for development and the preconditions for implementing them. The upcycling of sustainable knowledge that has *relevance* and *quality* can contribute to sound management, increase the surplus value of knowledge capital and prevent research waste (Malterud, 2019).

What will this book offer you?

When conducting a research project, your aim will determine which method is best suited to provide the answers you seek. By reading this book, you will learn about the hallmarks of the qualitative metasynthesis research method and how it developed. The book's outline follows a traditional research process, with planning, literature search, review and assessment of primary studies to be included in your sample, analysis and synthesis and, finally, reporting your project. In addition, you will be exposed to discussions about the scientific challenges that emerge when qualitative research methods encounter methodology from *evidence-based medicine* (EBM) (Malterud, 2019).

Several of the metasyntheses that you will find in the research litera-ture imply extensive efforts, with comprehensive searches, large num-bers of hits and screening procedures requiring significant resources. The format I have used and still prefer deals with the interpretation and analysis of a limited and thus feasible number of primary studies (Larun & Malterud, 2007; Malterud & Ulriksen, 2011; Dahl et al., 2013; Fosse et al., 2014). This format is not typical of today's qualitative metasyntheses, which often involve extensive searches. Throughout the book I therefore discuss the preconditions needed for this kind of research to be conducted sustainably, which choices will be encoun-tered and what the consequences of these choices may be. At the same time, I emphasize the idea that research should be feasible in practice, with accountable use of research resources.

To understand the messages of this book, you will need some basic knowledge of qualitative research methods. If you are a novice, you should therefore start by learning the fundamental methodological principles from an introductory textbook. A novice also needs a super-visor or collaborator with a general competence in qualitative research methods. Subsequently, you can together decide whether you want to conduct a qualitative primary study or to synthesize existing evidence about the problem under investigation. If you choose the latter course, you will realize that there are several paths to reach your goal. Using examples from my own and other researchers' publications, I present research questions where qualitative metasynthesis may be an appro-priate strategy. This book will show you different options and offer some practical recommendations.

The role of the nursing home doctor in end-of-life care – a concrete example

Most Norwegians spend their last period of life in a nursing home, however long that period may be (Statistics Norway, 2013). The nurs-ing home doctor (NHD) is responsible for the medical aspects of the stay, such as diagnosis, treatment and palliation of disease and loss of function. Their professional duties towards individuals in this life stage imply several existential, medical and organizational challenges. Sometimes, patients and relatives have distinct wishes and stand-points, while in other situations death can approach without impor-tant issues having been resolved. Dialogue between patients, relatives, caring professionals and the NHD during this stage is essential but not always easy to implement in a satisfactory manner (Aase et al., 2008; Jansen et al., 2016). To offer knowledge-based practice, we need an overview of the kind of research that can offer support and the results this research has provided.

Anette Fosse, who is a general practitioner and NHD in Mo i Rana in northern Norway, has long-time experience in end-of-life care. She wanted to conduct a research project as a contribution to her colleagues that would best support their encounters with this patient group. Fosse started exploring the relevant existing research about this topic by conducting a review of qualitative studies about end-of-life experiences and expectations among nursing home patients and their relatives (Fosse et al., 2014). She could have chosen to obtain an overview by means of a straightforward literature search. Instead, she took the opportunity to learn about meta-ethnography, one of the several available methods in qualitative metasynthesis (see Chapter 3) (Noblit & Hare, 1988). Fosse's project serves as an example throughout this book.

From chaos and individual research reports to systematic reviews

The international research literature has become nothing less than enormous, especially in recent decades. You will need relevant tools, competence and resources to establish a general idea of the research that is already there. You will also need methodical and professional insight to assess the relevance and quality of the reports you find. A literature review based on transparent identification, selection and synthesis of primary studies embodies the research methodology used to develop systematic reviews (SRs). Qualitative metasyntheses are often presented as a specific kind of SR that employs the synthesis of qualitative studies. There are, however, important issues to be reflected upon regarding such a conceptualization. Below, we therefore start the presentation of this method by laying out certain principles that underlie any SR, independent of the method used in the primary studies.

Comprehensive and critical reading of the research literature

Literature reviews and other articles in which the research literature about a question is presented and summarized are an established genre in the medical publication tradition. This format has long been comparatively casual, with the author's discretion prioritizing the publications that are selected and emphasized. My own publication list includes some articles of this kind. In hindsight, I must admit that my choice of references may have been motivated by a need to support my own arguments. Today, however, an acceptable *review article* should do more than just list previous knowledge – it should also offer an interpretation and appraisal of the evidence presented.

Scientific knowledge is supposed to be the outcome of systematic reflection as opposed to casual impressions or self-confirming arguments. This is also true of qualitative studies and of their syntheses (Malterud, 2001b). If I claim in the capacity of researcher that I have explored something, it is not acceptable to give a brief report about the first article that comes along. Qualitative research methods do not confer any authority to legitimize such superficial observations.

Knowledge, including overviews and upcycling of existing evidence, is always developed from a specific context that determines the perspectives and gazes of the researcher (Latour & Woolgar, 1986; Alvesson & Sköldberg, 2009; Saini & Shlonsky, 2012; Malterud, 2019). We read that research with our preconceptions and theoretical frames of references in mind, often with a tendency to focus our eyes on texts that confirm our own point of view (Kelly et al., 2015). *Reflexivity* is an active attitude, a position that the researcher must seek out and maintain (Malterud, 2002; Finlay, 2008). The skilful researcher establishes positions that challenge preconceptions and previous field knowledge, including searching and reading the existing literature.

Systematic knowledge management requires that the researcher makes the reader an informed companion who is given insight into the preconditions under which the knowledge has been developed (Malterud, 1993, 2001b; Stige et al., 2009). This is what we call *intersubjectivity*. A related academic ideal is *transparency*, which means that the process is visible to and can be contested by others. This kind of scientific presumption is applicable to all steps of the research process, not merely to the analysis of one's own empirical data or to qualitative research methods. When our aim is to develop a literature review with the status of a scientific project, we must proceed methodically and give the reader access to our procedures, assessments and choices. Specific research methods have been established for this purpose.

Qualitative metasynthesis is an overarching concept including research methods that enable the identification, review and synthesis of qualitative studies about different topics. Here, I shall refer to this concept as the process and outcome of organizing and interpreting research findings about a particular matter, leading to new, conceptual understanding beyond the average or sum of parts (Malterud, 2017a, 2019). Several procedures are available – the one we choose will be determined by what we want to explore and the analytic ambitions and resources of our project. Later in this book, you will read more about similarities in and differences between different methods of analysis. When the methodological rules of the game are followed, this kind of strategy leads to independent research offering new knowledge.

The information deluge

With the digital revolution and public accessibility to the internet in the 1990s, researchers all over the world could gain access to the international research literature with only a few keystrokes. On the one hand, this development unleashed a massive democratization of the knowledge base. In recent years, this trend has been further enhanced by the efforts to provide open access to research. However, access to large parts of the research literature is regulated by expensive subscription systems, leaving one effectively stranded if one has no connection to an academic institution with sufficient resources. On the other hand, the total volume of research literature has expanded greatly, to some extent of variable and unpredictable scientific quality. As a researcher, you will need adequate tools to navigate safely through this deluge of information. Professional assistance for the literature search will also be useful.

Sustainable management of the information deluge requires methods for upcycling and elaborating on existing research evidence. We start our pursuit with an identification and critical assessment of *primary studies*, which means individual empirical studies – whether qualitative, quantitative or a combination – that have already been published in peer-reviewed journals. These primary studies are used to create synopses, reviews or syntheses and to activate knowledge capital, making it possible to repay it with interest. For example, a qualitative primary study could involve a focus group of patients with obesity discussing their experiences in their encounters with general practitioners (Malterud & Ulriksen, 2010). An SR of a related topic could, for example, be a metasynthesis about stigma and obesity in the health care system (Malterud & Ulriksen, 2011).

Broad mapping

When entering a new field of research, we will often begin with a broad mapping of the literature to obtain an impression of the most common kind of research, the concepts that are used and the kind of knowledge that remains absent. In this way, we can also develop an image of the impact of different theoretical perspectives and of how previous research has been formed by different positions. This is useful when we identify our own motives and attitudes, hit upon our own point of departure, appraise concepts and definitions and position ourselves according to existing research (Finlay, 2008; Stige et al., 2009).

We may start with a rough mapping of the knowledge base without subsequent critical discussion of results or implications. These are often called *mapping studies* (Cooper, 2016). In these reviews, the studies identified in the literature search are usually not subjected to quality assessment. A test search or *scoping review* may offer a more compelling introduction to topics explored in articles of various and complex designs, especially when there is not an abundance of existing reviews (Arksey & O'Malley, 2005; The Joanna Briggs Institute, 2015). Colquhoun et al. (2014) emphasize that this kind of review is a new and hitherto rather messy tradition with inconsistent terminology and methodology and offer this definition:

> A scoping review or scoping study is a form of knowledge synthesis that addresses an exploratory research question aimed at mapping key concepts, types of evidence, and gaps in research related to a defined area or field by systematically searching, selecting, and synthesizing existing knowledge.

It is particularly useful to find out whether one or more high-quality SRs about your topic is already available. When such reviews exist, it is reasonable to elaborate on others' efforts instead of starting the process from scratch.

Systematic reviews – a specific kind of research literature summary

A *systematic review* (SR) is the outcome of a research literature summary conducted according to a particular research methodology. The aim is to map the landscape and present the existing relevant research evidence of proper quality within a certain field. When Fosse set out to plan her own primary study and develop an original and precise research aim about the role of the NHD in encounters with end-of-life patients, a comprehensive literature search would have constituted a useful and necessary point of departure. When she instead decided to make that literature review an independent research project by conducting a qualitative metasynthesis, she was confronted with more specific methodological criteria regarding process and outcome (Fosse et al., 2014).

The principles and procedures for these research literature summaries have been cultivated as a scientific method in EBM (Sackett et al., 1996).

The Cochrane Collaboration (Chalmers, 1993) expressed as an explicit aim that *evidence-based policy* would be supported by SRs that present an overarching summary of the status of research into a given question, and specific principles and methods were developed (Oxman & Guyatt, 1993; Lavis et al., 2005; Liberati et al., 2009; Gough et al., 2017b):

> Systematic Review: The application of strategies that limit bias in the assembly, critical appraisal, and synthesis of all relevant studies on a specific topic. Meta-analysis may be, but is not necessarily, used as part of this process.
>
> (O'Rourke, 2007)

Using the term SR has implications for both methodological premises and the final report, for both approach and result. The process includes clarifying the problem and question, finding, describing and synthesizing the relevant research literature, appraising the relevance and quality of the evidence and presenting and using the research findings (Gough et al., 2017a). Several checklists and other criteria for the quality assessment of primary studies have been developed (see Chapter 2). SRs imply the recycling and upcycling of individual primary studies, but the concept can also be applied to reviews of reviews – i.e., identifying, critically assessing and crafting a synopsis of previously presented SRs.

In Norway, the Division of Health Services in the Norwegian Institute of Public Health (previously the Norwegian Knowledge Centre for the Health Services, an independent government unit – NOKC) has been a leading institution for the development, application and promotion of this methodology. The centre has worked out a comprehensive SR manual (Nasjonalt kunnskapssenter for helsetjenesten, 2015). It advises that SRs of research evidence are distinguished by systematic and explicit procedures regarding how the research question is formulated, the procedures of the literature search and the assessment, synopsis and presentation of the subsequent research knowledge. NOKC requires the following criteria to be fulfilled for a review to qualify as systematic:

1   The review must be based on an explicit search strategy.
2   The review must contain well-defined inclusion criteria.
3   The primary studies or reviews included in the review must be assessed for methodical quality.

In brief, an SR implies not only a systematic approach but also a transparent strategy. Similar requirements are applicable to qualitative metasynthesis, where a comparable methodology is used for the sustainable identification, upcycling and synthesis of existing qualitative studies (Malterud, 2019). Moreover, this must be accomplished with due respect for the basic principles of qualitative research methods.

Evidence from research results

Medical and health care practices are based on knowledge from several different sources. Research results, clinical experience, qualified judgment and interaction all contribute to understanding health and disease and how these factors are perceived and can be influenced. Human experiences, values and priorities have a great impact on the priorities and emphasis placed on different sources of knowledge in general, in research specifically and in encounters with individuals. Research results are often called evidence, but what counts as evidence and how we assess its quality are both matters of extensive debate. In this chapter, we focus on concerns that determine which kinds of knowledge are regarded as valid and useful under different circumstances.

Multipurpose knowledge capital

Evidence denotes "the available body of facts or information indicating whether a belief or proposition is true or valid" (Oxford English Dictionary). The concept means something different in everyday language ("there was no obvious evidence of a break-in") than in more formal contexts as information used to establish facts in a legal investigation or admissible as testimony in a law court (Oxford English Dictionary). While the first connotation may suggest that further proofs are not necessary, the second connotation points towards scientific or legal knowledge, with its associations with the natural sciences, testing hypotheses and deductive strategies, all leading to facts or truths. In this book, I use the word *evidence* as an overarching term for research results, independent of topic, method or quality. Hence, there are many kinds of evidence, each developed for different purposes with diverse strategies and possessing varying levels of quality (Malterud, 2019).

In taking a closer look at the medical traditions regarding knowledge, we find an interesting contradiction between ideals and realities. On the one hand, the positivist foundation of biomedicine indicates that medical knowledge is supposed to be the outcome of natural science research, in order to secure generalizability. On the other hand, clinical practice indicates that substantial proportions of this practice domain actually rest on tacit, experience-based knowledge (Malterud, 1995, 2001a). A patient's history is for example the most important source of a doctor's diagnostic judgments (Peterson et al., 1992). Montgomery describes this incongruity as rational, research-based practice in which the discipline idolizes a simplified and old-fashioned version of science (Montgomery, 2006).

Several similar paradoxes occur regularly in medical and health care services theory and practice. Their existence offers good arguments for breadth as to sources of knowledge, research methods and types of evidence, especially regarding the impact of qualitative research methods, systematic reflection on experiences from clinical practice and the importance of interaction, context and values (Malterud, 2001a, 2001b). I do not argue that one is better than the other but insist that we need a diversity of knowledge and research results to understand patients, diseases and health care systems. It is far from obvious that evidence is most valid when expressed in numerical terms. The research question will determine what kind of answer is best.

For SRs, we may address incoming and outgoing evidence. *Incoming evidence* is the documentation and results from primary studies that we apply as a point of departure for analysis and synthesis, while *outgoing evidence* is the outcome of this process (Malterud, 2019). The quality of outgoing evidence is closely connected to the quality of incoming evidence and of the methodology used for elaboration. Still, the quality of outgoing evidence cannot be assessed without considering the context of application for the outgoing evidence (see Chapter 4).

Evidence-based medicine

EBM was established to replace clinical impressions, anecdotal experiences, expert opinions and tradition with scientific evidence as the foundation for health care decisions (Levin, 2001; Smith & Rennie, 2014). Sackett et al. (1996) emphasize that this was not intended to constrain the definition of types of knowledge or evidence:

> Evidence based medicine is the conscientious, explicit, and judicious use of current best evidence in making decisions about the care of individual patients.

For this purpose, the Cochrane Collaboration developed guidelines for putting together SRs (Liberati et al., 2009; Cochrane Collaboration, 2011). Initially this methodology was created to summarize studies about the effects of medical interventions, primarily based on *randomized controlled trials* (*RCTs*). Gradually, similar principles were also used as a basis for review of other kinds of medical and health services research.

Today, SRs include much more than effect studies. NOKC and other Cochrane-affiliated institutions have published SRs about diagnosis and screening, disease prevention and psychosocial programs and different kinds of health services, in addition to summaries and syntheses of classic effect studies on drug treatments or vaccines (Malterud et al., 2016a). Software and manuals for SRs of studies about diagnostic tests have been developed, such as the quality assessment of diagnostic accuracy studies (*QUADAS*) (Whiting et al., 2011), which was established to standardize questions about patient samples, the test to be examined, the gold standard for that test and the process for examining the test.

Different research questions require different evidence from relevant methodologies

Several authors have argued that the EBM model for SRs is insufficient to summarize research knowledge about health and health services in general. In particular, health services researchers trained in social sciences have demanded that effect studies must be complemented with evidence with the capacity to say more about the contextual, political and ethical preconditions and consequences of the evidence (Black, 2001; Mays et al., 2005; Orton et al., 2011; Greenhalgh, 2012; Gough et al., 2017a).

A principal aspect of this debate deals with the knowledge base itself. In clinical encounters, doctors synthesize evidence available from different paradigms and sources (Malterud, 2001a). What actually constitutes evidence and other valid sources of knowledge for medicine and health care? Is research the only and most important source of evidence? Which areas of the practice field require other kinds of research-based knowledge than the outcomes of effect studies designed as RCTs? How can such matters be explored in a relevant and trustworthy way?

Greenhalgh et al. (2014) argue that

> real evidence based medicine has the care of individual patients as its top priority, asking, 'what is the best course of action for this patient, in these circumstances, at this point in their illness or condition?' It consciously and reflexively refuses to let process (doing tests, prescribing medicines) dominate outcomes (the agreed goal

of management in an individual case). It engages with an ethical and existential agenda (how should we live? when should we accept death?) and with that goal in mind, carefully distinguishes between whether to investigate, treat, or screen and how to do so.

I have also engaged in such debates. My experiences as a general practitioner over several decades have convinced me that only a limited number of the clinical activities in the practice domain are accessible by or suitable for effect studies (Malterud, 1995, 2001a). At the same time, I realized with increasing clarity that diversity in epistemology and methodology would be necessary to draw attention to clinical knowledge in a systematic and transparent way, although without dismissing quantitative studies when they could offer useful evidence. To me, purposeful relevance became a significant concept to reflect on what we regard as evidence and how we assess its quality. Consequently, I have, over the years in several different circumstances, argued that qualitative research methods can offer useful and valid evidence about medical problems (Malterud, 2001b, 2002, 2016).

An extensive number of qualitative studies dealing with individuals' perceptions and experiences with health, illness and health care encounters have been published. These results represent a broad range of evidence of different types and qualities. In the last decades we have also witnessed an increasing number of SRs in which evidence from qualitative studies is summarized and synthesized (Tong et al., 2012; Thorne, 2017). Sustainable upcycling can broaden and enrich our sense of knowledge and evidence while making it more contested.

At the Cochrane Collaboration, an increasing understanding developed that evidence from SRs of high-quality RCTs might have important limitations when used as the basis for decisions in practice and policy – an essential objective for literature reviews in this tradition. Evidence regarding the feasibility, acceptability and values related to the health care intervention has been called for (Schünemann et al., 2006; Lewin et al., 2018). Several authors argue that qualitative studies could contribute to reviews of complex interventions by shifting attention to what is going on and how it developed instead of asking solely about efficacy.

In 2006, the Cochrane Collaboration established a working group to develop guidelines for the integration of evidence from qualitative studies in SRs about the effect of interventions (Hannes et al., 2013). A specific chapter about qualitative evidence in the *Cochrane Handbook of Systematic Review of Interventions* first appeared in 2008 and has since been revised several times (Noyes et al., 2015).

This methodology, known as *qualitative evidence synthesis*, is steadily being elaborated. This research environment has contributed to the World Health Organization's decision to accept qualitative studies as evidence in complex interventions (Glenton et al., 2016a). Still, SRs of qualitative studies are often referred to as supplemental to traditional SRs of effect studies (Saini & Shlonsky, 2012).

From summary and renarration to interpretation and synthesis

When crafting an SR, we identify knowledge that has the potential for further elaboration and interpretation. Our task is not only to summarize the knowledge we identify but also to use analysis and synthesis to develop independent results and new evidence. The sustainable upcycling of relevant evidence of appropriate quality leads to a growth in knowledge capital. Our research questions, ambitions, competences and available resources will determine whether it is possible to aim for a level of analysis at which synthesis can be conducted. In this respect, incoming evidence from the primary studies must have enough information power for proper interpretation to offer something novel.

Descriptive, interpretative or both?

An SR without statistical analysis will often present its results as an epic story, without extensive analysis or elaboration. This is usually called a *narrative summary* or *review* (Snilstveit et al., 2012) –an unfortunate and misleading concept too easily confused with *narrative analysis* of qualitative data, a specific qualitative methodological tradition based on literary science (Riessman, 2008; Josselson, 2011; Frank, 2012). Narrative analysis offers tools for systematic exploration of the meaning in texts presenting narratives. Roles, structure, temporality and plot are the principal dimensions in the analysis of narratives, which is completely different from what is emphasized in what are called narrative reviews. Dixon-Woods et al. (2005) argue, moreover, that narrative reviews represent a less binding format that suffers from low levels of transparency.

SRs include not only identification, summary and recapitulation of primary studies but also a systematic critical assessment, reanalysis and synthesis of the incoming as well as the outgoing evidence (Gough et al., 2017a). The methodological literature differentiates between two types of reviews: *descriptive* or *aggregative reviews,* in which existing knowledge is collected and added up, and *interpretative* or *configurative reviews,* in which evidence from existing research is elaborated, reanalysed and configured (Thorne, 2015; Gough et al., 2017a). The two formats share a systematic and transparent strategy for the literature search and subsequent sorting and assessment, while analysis and summing up are accomplished in different ways (Malterud, 2019).

Qualitative metasynthesis is supposed to have an interpretative ambition beyond renarrration. This book emphasizes interpretative SRs, with a goal of accomplishing a synthesis leading to something else and something more than the individual studies included in the review. Selecting the appropriate theoretical perspectives are useful to support this kind of analysis (Malterud, 2016).

Meta-analysis

Meta-analysis is a method of summarizing and reanalysing evidence from already published primary studies to answer a joint research question:

> Meta-Analysis: The statistical synthesis of the data from separate but similar, i.e. comparable studies, leading to a quantitative summary of the pooled results.
>
> (O'Rourke, 2007)

This concept was initially presented in the late 1970s to summarize effect estimates from different primary studies using comparable interventions. A classic example deals with calculating the effect of aspirin on secondary prevention of myocardial infarction (Editorial Lancet, 1980). Meta-analysis can provide statistical power by compiling several small studies, thereby offering a more reliable overall picture. This strategy implies that the primary studies have measured the same outcomes with a comparable method in comparable samples of participants and have not merely investigated the same research question.

It is often assumed that meta-analysis means statistical analysis. Still, it is possible to imagine meta-analyses of qualitative or quantitative primary studies or even both (mixed methods, see Chapter 4), with various levels of ambition as to synthesis. Nevertheless, a critical assessment of the included primary studies regarding relevance and quality must be conducted, and an adequate methodology for synopsis must be adopted. An important difference is that quantitative meta-analysis uses the data from the primary studies as the basis for analysis, while qualitative meta-analysis uses the results from the primary studies in analysis and synthesis (Sandelowski, 2012).

By means of its connection to the Cochrane Collaboration, the NOKC has developed competence and contributed to the implementation of methods for SRs in health services research and policy (Jamtvedt, 2013; Mørland, 2014; Nasjonalt kunnskapssenter for helsetjenesten). The assignment from the authorities has been to provide SRs with meta-analysis as the basis for decision-making in health care. Still, the development of new knowledge can be an independent objective in academic practice, different from the Cochrane objective of guideline development. Relevance is always an important criterion for scientific quality, but SRs are not always initiated by a commission related to policy decisions or pointed in a particular applied direction.

Several research environments inside and outside the EBM tradition demonstrate an increasing understanding of the knowledge impact of qualitative studies and of SRs of such studies (Glenton et al., 2013). To a certain extent, these approaches address some of the limitations of the traditional Cochrane methodology for SRs of quantitative primary studies (Guyatt et al., 2011; Petticrew, 2015). Nevertheless, summarized quantitative effect studies constitute a huge majority among the SRs from NOKC (Malterud et al., 2016a).

Qualitative metasynthesis

The methodological foundation for the summary, upcycling and synthesis of qualitative studies was developed in the 1980s, independent of the Cochrane Collaboration efforts (Thorne et al., 2004; Sandelowski & Barroso, 2007). As early as 1985, Stern and Harris published an article that synthesized the main findings of seven different primary studies about women and self-care (Stern & Harris, 1985). Noblit and Hare (1988) presented *meta-ethnography* as a method for synthesizing the findings of qualitative studies for analysis and interpretation, not just for summing up. The authors pointed out that their method differed from quantitative meta-analysis, in which the data from primary studies are integrated (see Chapter 3 for more about meta-ethnography). This strategy enjoyed widespread approval and use, also for the synthesis of different types of qualitative studies without a specifically ethnographic foundation (Dixon-Woods et al., 2006; Bondas & Hall, 2007b). Later, several other types of SRs and meta-analyses of qualitative studies beyond meta-ethnography were presented (see Chapter 3).

Qualitative research methods belong to the interpretative paradigm (see Chapter 4) in which subjectivity and meaning are recognized and explored, with the researcher as an integral and participating tool (Malterud, 2016). In a qualitative study, the researcher applies descriptions and interpretation. It is not possible to have one without the other, since any description is affected by interpretations, and any interpretation takes descriptions as a point of departure. To be sure, there are realist positioned qualitative studies where the researcher's explicit ambition is to describe reality as accurately as possible. Yet, most qualitative research methods resonate with a social constructionist understanding that the world can be perceived in different ways depending on the position one takes and the perspectives one chooses (Lock & Strong, 2010). This is not to say that everything is relative and fluent – we realize that interpretations from other researchers can win (or fail to win) approval and be regarded as meaningful (or dismissed) by others. Sandelowski (2012) presents sensible arguments for such an epistemological standpoint, which may be conceptualized as *subtle realism*.

Interpretation is a methodological hallmark of all kinds of qualitative studies, which is also inherent in summaries and syntheses of qualitative primary studies like qualitative metasyntheses. The analysis is assumed to lead towards a new understanding beyond a literal recapitulation of what was previously said and written (Noblit & Hare, 1988). Campbell et al. expressed this ambition as follows:

> Synthesis of qualitative research can be envisaged as the bringing together of findings on a chosen theme, the results of which should, in conceptual terms, be greater than the sum of parts. Thus, the purpose of a qualitative synthesis would be to achieve greater understanding and attain a level of conceptual or theoretical development beyond that achieved in any individual empirical study.
>
> (Campbell et al., 2003)

The research literature presents different concepts for summary and analysis of qualitative primary studies. While some write about qualitative research synthesis (Major & Savin-Baden, 2010), others use the term qualitative evidence synthesis (Lewin et al., 2015; Booth, 2016). Below, we emphasize the hallmarks, strengths and challenges of the qualitative methods for the presentation and discussion of SRs of qualitative studies.

For this book, I have chosen the concept *qualitative metasynthesis* to highlight a position of interpretation, inductive analysis and synthesis as major requirements for the development of new knowledge about subjectivity and meaning (Noblit & Hare, 1988; Major & Savin-Baden, 2010; Sandelowski, 2012; Thorne, 2017), based on sustainable incoming evidence characterized by relevance and quality (Malterud, 2019). The number of published qualitative metasyntheses has increased every year, especially in the last decade (Tong et al., 2012). Much of this growth is due to calls for SRs (including, slowly but surely, also qualitative studies) from policymakers at different levels (Glenton et al., 2016a). Another hypothesis to explain this increase is that the SR methodology has been elaborated and become more robust, so that qualitative metasynthesis is now an approved and independent research method.

Fosse (2014) struggled to understand how medical effect studies would provide useful and relevant knowledge about the role of the NHD at the end of life. This topic involved processes, interaction and existential matters rather than effects and efficacy. Fosse had already come across several interesting qualitative studies about this topic. She began to wonder whether it would be possible to summarize existing research evidence in a sustainable way, striving for new knowledge with the capacity to make a difference for clinical practice.

Which kinds of research questions can be studied with qualitative metasynthesis?

Qualitative metasynthesis can be used to sum up all kinds of qualitative primary studies and is consequently suited to explore the kind of research questions where qualitative research methods are appropriate. Metasynthesis may expand our knowledge about individuals' experiences, practices, thoughts, expectations, motives and attitudes. We can pursue the meaning, impact and nuances of events and behaviour, and we can strengthen our understanding of why people act as they do, given their social, cultural and historical conditions. Qualitative methods, including metasyntheses, are not appropriate strategies when prevalence, distribution, effects or other quantitative outcome measures are on the menu. Furthermore, the aim is not to repeat or confirm existing evidence but to apply that knowledge to the development of new evidence and understanding.

Qualitative metasynthesis can help us upcycle knowledge capital to gain insights into individuals' experiences with different diseases, living conditions or treatment programs, such as prostate cancer and ethnicity (Rivas et al., 2016), multiple sclerosis and exercise treatment (Christensen et al., 2016), isolation in stem cell transplantation (Biagioli et al., 2016), diabetes and self-care (Campbell et al., 2003) or quality of life in dementia (O'Rourke et al., 2015). How do children experience a childhood with parents who suffer from serious mental illness (Dam & Hall, 2016)? What kinds of strain do military families undergo due to repeated relocation (Yablonsky et al., 2016)? Which stigmas do people with obesity experiences when they encounter health care services (Malterud & Ulriksen, 2011)?

Several metasyntheses deal with individuals' understanding of and practices in the use of medication, such as treatment of tuberculosis or asthma (Britten et al., 2002; Atkins et al., 2008; Britten & Pope, 2011). This research method can also be used to further the development of knowledge about the health care experiences of different groups of patients, such as patients with Chronic fatigue syndrome/Myalgic encephalopathy (CFS/ME) (Larun & Malterud, 2007; Anderson et al., 2011), lesbian couples encountering the maternity ward (Dahl et al., 2013) or those presenting with early cancer symptoms (Smith et al., 2005).

When we want to explore experiences or preconditions for practices and attitudes among health care providers, existing research findings – sometimes also including existing metasyntheses – can provide a point of departure. Among these are metasyntheses about general practitioners' attitudes about guidelines (Carlsen et al., 2007) or about medically unexplained symptoms (Johansen & Risor, 2016), conditions for safety voices in health care workplaces (Morrow et al., 2016), practices among mental health care nurses regarding patients with personality disorders (Dickens et al., 2016), knowledge sources used by newly graduated nurses (Voldbjerg et al., 2016) and experiences among oncologists of breaking bad news to patients (Bousquet et al., 2015).

Studies of community health problems related to disease prevention and health-promoting programs may also be summed up using metasynthesis, such as the preconditions for condom use among Asian sex workers (Tan & Melendez-Torres, 2016) or communication from public health authorities to the population during pandemics (Carlsen & Glenton, 2016).

Still, neither a relevant topic nor a lack of existing knowledge is enough to initiate or complete a qualitative metasynthesis. When Fosse (2014) started considering whether this method could be appropriate for her aim of developing new knowledge about the role of the NHD at the end of life, she also had to assess the likelihood that there were a sufficient number of sustainable primary studies to use for further analysis. Moreover, she would have to craft a sufficiently focused research question to properly manage and review a feasible number of hits from the literature search. Finally, her research team had to consider whether they possessed the appropriate qualitative methodological skills and whether the available resources of time, human infrastructure and assistance would be appropriate. Unless these issues were resolved satisfactorily, it would have been better to plan a different kind of study about the topic.

2 Project planning and literature management

Careful preparations are profitable investments

Thorough planning is necessary to ensure your project's feasibility and quality. To reach your goal and develop evidence that makes new and useful insights available, you must craft a strategy and work out a detailed and specific protocol. Several principles and procedures that are part of a qualitative metasynthesis are comparable to any research project, including qualitative primary studies and quantitative SRs. However, qualitative metasynthesis is a specific methodology that requires preparations and skills regarding data collection and analysis, not least because there are different paths to reaching the goal. Let us take a closer look at some of the preliminary preparations.

Summing up research – a stepwise process

The research process of a qualitative metasynthesis can be described with the same principal pattern as for any SR. To be sure, analysis and synthesis are vital elements of the research process which you must consider thoroughly and specifically when planning your project. They do not appear by themselves, and it is not obvious which choices will best serve your project.

Below, you will find an overview of issues to consider when planning a qualitative metasynthesis (Oliver et al., 2012; Saini & Shlonsky, 2012; Gough et al., 2017a). You should not do this planning on your own the first time you embark on such a project. If you do not have ample experience with this method, you will need assistance from your supervisor or collaborators in preparing and carrying out the project. At this point, we take for granted that you have already invested the time and resources needed to become acquainted with the topic, made yourself familiar with the terminology and developed a focused research question. You must also take the time needed to gain knowledge of the method of your choice.

The issues below are described in more detail in subsequent chapters.

- Research question
- Literature search
    - Initial overview; elaborate wording of research question
    - Collaboration with research librarian about search words and search strategy
    - Test search followed by ultimate literature search
- Review and selection of potential primary studies – make flowsheet
    - Management of references
    - Exclusion of duplicates
    - Screening the hits (title and abstract) regarding relevance, adjusting and documentation of criteria along the way
    - Assess relevance of candidate articles (full text)
    - Decide on criteria for quality assessment and implement them with the remaining candidate articles
- Overview of included primary studies
    - Develop procedures for practical management of the primary studies included
    - Detailed reading of the primary studies included, organize important features in a table
    - Data extraction with identification and organization of results from the primary studies
- Analysis and synthesis
    - Accomplish management of data, analysis and synthesis according to the method and theoretical perspective chosen
- Accounting for the evidence
    - Synthesize major findings
    - Present the results and write an article

A research question that is both flexible and determined

Before you decide on methods and procedures, you must take the time to elaborate and refine your research question, considering why and how your strategy may make a difference. It is a good idea to invite some respected colleagues to engage in a collective effort to clarify, challenge and improve your research question as much as possible. Afterwards, you can better decide on the design that offers the best possibilities to explore your particular question. Do not initiate the process with a predetermined conclusion to accomplish a qualitative metasynthesis – perhaps an empirical primary study will turn up to be better suited for what you want to find out about, or perhaps a straightforward survey.

The probability that a qualitative metasynthesis will help us find our way through the enormous jungle of existing research literature increases to the extent that we know specifically what it is we are investigating. A thoroughly prepared research question is therefore a crucial precondition for a successful outcome. We do not, however, use this question for hypothesis testing, as we would in a quantitative study (Petticrew, 2015).

The best research question is sufficiently flexible to approach most of the research literature within the area we want to explore. At the same time, it is specific enough for our synthesis to contribute something new rather than simply presenting a catalogue of what is already known. The challenge is to find an adequate balance between these standards (Atkins et al., 2008). If we set out too broad and general, we run a substantial risk of drowning in literature references and losing our way. For example, in her study about the nursing home doctor's (NHD's) role, Fosse emphasized expectations and experiences from patients and relatives and decided not to cover research about the experiences of doctors or nursing professionals (Fosse et al., 2014).

Eakin and Mykhalovskiy (2003) argue that a qualitative study's research question is more like a compass than an anchor and therefore is often not finalized until the last part of the research process. For this reason, in any qualitative study we should revise the research question during the process as we learn more about which kind of knowledge the empirical data will allow us to flesh out (Malterud, 2019).

The research question is expressed as a short sentence in which you articulate as specifically as possible what you want to know more about. Include neither issues related to motivation and overarching goal (which belong in the introductory paragraphs of your protocol and article) nor details about how you intend to accomplish the metasynthesis (which belong in the methods section). Fosse (2014) writes that the aim of her study was to identify and synthesize qualitative research findings about nursing home patients' and their relatives' expectations and experiences of how doctors can contribute to quality end-of-life care.

Choosing a strategy

There are several strategies available for conducting a qualitative metasynthesis (Noblit & Hare, 1988; Dixon-Woods et al., 2005; Bondas & Hall,

2007b; Barnett-Page & Thomas, 2009; Kastner et al., 2016; Finfgeld-Connett, 2018). The differences among them involve the literature search, the selection of studies to be included and the quality assessment of the primary studies. There are also different methods for analysis and synthesis and different strategies for the application of theoretical perspectives during the analysis. You will have to make yourself sufficiently familiar with the various methodologies to make an informed choice of procedure which you will be able to follow correctly and defend later on. These recommendations apply to principles, procedures and terminology. Do not try to combine several different methods unless you are very experienced, capable to describe, explain and justify your path.

Across most strategies for qualitative metasynthesis, we notice a stepwise procedure that recalls Noblit and Hare's seven-step model for meta-ethnography (1988). This model also bears resemblances to the general principles of qualitative analysis. Here, we emphasize similarities in procedure, irrespective of strategy. Chapter 3 offers a more detailed presentation of meta-ethnography and a brief presentation of some other common methods for analysis.

The protocol

Crafting a thorough research protocol will help you to clarify your thoughts and focus your efforts, whether you are a novice or already have skills and experiences in qualitative metasynthesis. When writing the protocol, you constrain yourself to prepare your study in a logical way and to specify ideas and strategies. You are encouraged to concentrate your thoughts in a format that can be shared and contested. Reflexivity and interpretation throughout the project will be strengthened in a team of researchers with a wide range of professional and methodological skills and experiences.

The background section will demonstrate that you are already familiar with the basic research literature about your topic, thereby serving as a convincing argument for why the knowledge base lacks precisely what your metasynthesis will provide. A focused research question will determine whether the project will become valuable and feasible, standing out from what we already know well enough. A specific and realistic presentation of your method will assure your funders that the project is practicable and has sufficient validity.

The presentation of your work schedule, supervisory and collaborative relationships, funding, publication plan and list of references are also important elements of the protocol. In addition, the protocol for a qualitative metasynthesis should include explicit statements about the strategy for quality assessment of primary studies and available resources like library support, digital access to full-text research articles and considerations about ethical issues and privacy protection.

Your protocol can be a dynamic document which you adjust throughout the process as your research offers you experiences and helpful modifications. You should therefore update the protocol regularly, as if you were to submit it again in the following month. You can assign each new protocol a new name with a version number or date. As a rule, decisive adjustments can also be included in your decision trail. Summing up the project's status in this way will enhance the intersubjectivity of your project, and an updated protocol will help you share your progress with others. In addition, you have a text prepared in case new possibilities for presenting your project or obtaining funding should arise.

Registration of the project

To prevent unnecessary duplication, the NOKC recommends that any SR be registered in a central database (Nasjonalt kunnskapssenter for helsetjenesten, 2015). For qualitative metasyntheses, the *PROSPERO* database could be relevant (International prospective register of systematic reviews: https://www.crd.york.ac.uk/PROSPERO/). You should, however, be aware that this database was primarily established for SRs of effect studies. During registration, you will be asked several questions which are not relevant or possible to answer in connection with a qualitative metasynthesis. When answering the questions, remain faithful to the principles of the inductive process of an interpretative research method, where several types of decisions should be taken along the way with due consideration of the course of the process. Do not let yourself be locked up in advance by your answers at the registration stage.

Literature search

The results from the primary studies that we decide, item by item, to include for analysis constitute the empirical data for our qualitative metasynthesis. Methodological principles and specific procedures are different in this kind of data collection than in an empirical qualitative primary study, where the data might be transcripts from semi-structured individual interviews, to cite but one example. Our sample, consisting of the primary studies included, is not a casual collection but the endpoint of a systematic and transparent process developed specifically for this purpose. At the outset, we establish an overview of what has already been published about this or related topics. This overview is our point of departure for planning and implementing a comprehensive and methodical literature search.

Overview and steady course

A systematic literature search will counteract skewness by the selection of studies, so that we end up with something better than a map of the research literature that merely confirms our own ideas of what is important (Centre for Reviews and Disssemination, 2008). Booth (2016) presents three criteria for an effective search strategy: (i) it retrieves relevant records, (ii) it does not retrieve irrelevant references and (iii) the search terms as a whole are parsimonious to avoid redundancy.

It is often argued that the researcher in a qualitative study should set out broadly to obtain data beyond what was imagined as adequate in advance. In one way, this is true – we do not want to hinder our entrance to the field by assuming that we already know exactly what we will find. However, this is something other than a deliberate strategy to articulate what we want to explore. That is precisely why we conduct a systematic literature search – we hope and believe that we will find something we did not know in advance. My own experience is that all kinds of qualitative studies are enhanced by thorough preparations of this type far more than they would be by taking a general, non-specific route.

Some researchers warn against reading too much before you set out. Again, the challenge is to find an adequate level of preparation. You will not be able to develop new and sustainable knowledge without some idea of what others have already presented. In addition, you will not be able to establish relevant search terms without knowing what other researchers call the phenomena you want to explore. On the other hand, it is not wise to anticipate the SR while you are establishing an initial impression of the research literature in question – if you do, you will create unnecessary duplication of effort, and your preconceptions may come to override your systematic approaches.

A distinct and thoroughly prepared focus contributes to a steady course and prevents your metasynthesis from becoming simply a repetition of general matters about topics that are indeed important but do not offer anything substantially new (Sandelowski, 2012). In Fosse's study (2014) a search for studies about health care at the end of life, without further specification, would likely have led to innumerable references about terminal care, and a substantial part of the hits could only be used for exclusion as to relevance to the research question. Dahl et al. (2013), meanwhile, decided to concentrate their search for experiences among lesbian families encountering the maternity ward by excluding experiences with pregnancy care outside of hospital from their research question. With such strategies, it is possible to focus on the most relevant issues instead of searching too widely.

The research question determines which design you will prefer in primary studies assessed as relevant for inclusion. When intending to sum up research about individuals' experiences or practices, we search for qualitative primary studies rather than RCTs. If, on the other hand, our question deals with how many people suffer from a disease or a problem, a survey or a cross-sectional study may be adequate, while cohort studies can predict what will probably happen to patients with a particular disease. For a qualitative metasynthesis, the research question must comply with the relevant data from qualitative primary studies.

Search strategy

The classic version of the SR was developed in the evidence-based medicine (EBM) tradition to answer questions about which interventions are working and to contribute to improving the bases for decision-making in health care. The methodology was tailored for summing up studies about the effects of different interventions, most often RCTs. This point of departure is reflected in the acronym *PICO* (population–intervention–comparison–outcome), which is often recommended as a starting point to articulate the research question in an SR (Higgins & Green, 2011). The purpose of a qualitative metasynthesis is, however, to interpret and systematize knowledge about human and social phenomena and not to calculate effects, so we need not feel beholden to the PICO formula (Booth, 2016). Still, we can employ and translate some of its keywords to clarify our research question, as for example elaborated by Jamtvedt (2013):

- *Population*: Which kind of patient group?
    - What is the communal target group, main problems or diseases addressed in the primary studies we want to summarize?
- *Interventions*: Which actions?
    - Which kind of traits or experiences among the target group do we specifically want to explore?
- *Comparison*: Which settings to highlight?
    - Which social and cultural contexts do we want to emphasize when taking a closer look at this topic?

- *Outcome*: What to accomplish?
  - Do we also approach causal factors, conditions or consequences of the phenomena we study, beyond exploring experiences or expectations?

An alternative to PICO which has been developed for literature search in the synthesis of qualitative studies is *SPIDER* (sample, phenomenon of interest, design, evaluation, research type) (Cooke et al., 2012).

Your search strategy must be developed to accord with the research question you have articulated. For a classical SR based on quantitative studies with standardized designs, it makes sense to keep the research question and search strategy unchanged during the research process. In qualitative metasynthesis, on the other hand, we apply inductive and iterative strategies for which it will be more methodically appropriate to move three steps forward and two steps back to adjust our course as data collection, analysis and theoretical perspectives offer unexpected knowledge and new insights (see Chapter 4).

For example, these principles could imply that we concentrate on a purposive selection of the references we have identified in our search or that we complement our sample with relevant articles, perhaps backchaining from the reference lists in the included primary studies. Often, it will also be appropriate to adjust the research question to clarify what we are exploring. Still, we will rarely come to repeat our literature search from scratch as a consequence of such adjustments. The literature search is therefore an important effort deserving thorough preparation. The search strategy includes the choice and combination of search terms and the selection of bibliographic databases using appropriate time periods and languages of publication.

Search terms in logical combinations

Choosing precise search terms and combining them intelligently are necessary to conduct a literature search with the capacity to identify the most relevant primary studies for your topic. Most research literature is written in English, and search terms should therefore be in English, independent of your own native language. A useful initial manoeuvre is taking a close look at what you already have. When you have established an impression of the area, you will likely have a nice batch of quite casually selected articles about different aspects of the topic you want to approach in your qualitative metasynthesis. Make sure to note which keywords the article authors have used.

One primary study in Fosse's metasynthesis about the role of the NHD at the end of life (2014) dealt with issues emphasized by nursing home patients when establishing an advance care plan (ACP) that outlines the patient's end-of-life preferences (Lambert et al., 2005). In their article, the authors listed the following keywords:

> End of life; Advance care planning; Theoretical model; Grounded theory.

Next, you can look into how the article has been *indexed* in a major literature database, such as PubMed (https://www.ncbi.nlm.nih.gov/pubmed/). Here you will find the official keywords used in such databases, as listed for example in the medical subject headings classification system. For the ACP article, these keywords (abbreviated MH) were listed:

- *MH – Advance Directives/*psychology*
- *MH – Aged*
- *MH – Aged, 80 and over*
- *MH – Canada*
- *MH – *Decision Making*
- *MH – Fear*
- *MH – Female*
- *MH – Health Planning Guidelines*
- *MH – *Homes for the Aged*
- *MH – Humans*
- *MH – Information Dissemination*
- *MH – Long-Term Care*
- *MH – Male*
- *MH – *Nursing Homes*
- *MH – Social Support*
- *MH – Spirituality*

This list demonstrates why standardized keywords may lead to low precision from the perspective of research questions and results from qualitative primary studies. The indexing of qualitative studies in traditional medical databases is often insufficient and faulty, leading to an inadequate overview of existing research if traditional data sources and keywords are our only route of access (Grant, 2004; Tong et al., 2012; Booth, 2016). If your study deals with a topic that is not on the beaten medical path, such as a study about Chronic fatigue syndrome/Myalgic encephalopathy (CFS/ME) (Larun & Malterud, 2007), you will probably realize that the terminology in the research literature is inconsistent, muddy and even inaccurate. In such cases, wisely chosen significant expressions from the text of an article, especially from the abstract, may constitute a more successful *textword* search.

The authors of the ACP primary study, for example, expressed their aim as follows (Lambert et al., 2005):

> The purpose of this study was to describe factors contributing to the decision-making processes of elderly persons as they formulate advance directives in long-term care.

An experienced research librarian can help establish a rewarding search strategy based on the preparations described above. Professional library skills are also useful to develop logical combinations of search terms with *operators* such as AND, OR and NOT. You will also benefit from assistance in introducing search terms with different closing expressions, such as «emotion$», which includes both the singular and the plural forms. This is called *truncation*.

The outcome of this process in Fosse's meta-ethnography was presented as follows:

Text words entered individually, in combination, in full spelling and truncated:

> death; dying; end-of-life; palliative; terminal; nursing home; home for the aged; expectation; wish; fear; anxiety; forecasting; living will; advance directive; emotion; hope; perception; attitude to death; attitude to health; attitude to life; end-of-life experience; experience.
>
> (Fosse et al., 2014)

You can make your search strategy even more precise by adding different filters, such as those regarding methodology. Fosse decided to filter out any studies not conducted with a qualitative design. A similar strategy was chosen in a metasynthesis about stigma and obesity in the health care system (Malterud & Ulriksen, 2011).

Search sources and databases

Bibliographical databases are our most important sources for systematic literature searches. An experienced research librarian can help you find and select the most relevant databases. Prioritizing the different databases may be easier after you have had a dialogue about the research question and angle of the study you are planning; *Medline* and *CINAHL* tend to stand out as the databases with the best coverage for qualitative studies about health and disease (Booth, 2016). Your search should include neither too much nor too little – we try to balance the optimal level of *specificity* with the optimal level of *sensitivity* (Sandelowski, 2012). More than one database will usually be needed to achieve a search of sufficient scope. Some databases, on the other hand, may actually increase the proportion of contamination, leading to undesirably low specificity.

We will also have to decide how far back in time we want to search. On one hand, there are arguments for prioritizing more recent studies, which often have better methodological quality than older studies. On the other hand, historical results may help elucidate the research question. This was Dahl et al.'s experience in their metasynthesis about lesbian families encountering the maternity ward (2013) where a primary study from 1984 turned out to demonstrate interesting results that led to important historical contrasts in the analysis. Thorne (2017) emphasizes the impact of involving historical lines in the research literature; in the discussion paragraphs, we can often find the footprints of dialogues between researchers working at different points of time.

Below is a list of the seven bibliographical databases and the time span reviewed in Fosse's metasynthesis (2014):

* *Medline (Ovid) 1946 to September 17, 2012*
* *EMBASE (Ovid) 1974 to October 8, 2012*
* *PsycINFO (Ovid) 1806 to week 4 of September 2012*
* *CINAHL (Ebsco) 1981 to October 8, 2012*
* *Ageline (Ebsco) 1978 to October 8, 2012*
* *Cochrane Systematic Reviews (Wiley) Issue 9 of 12, September 2012*
* *Cochrane Trials (Wiley) Issue 9 of 12, September 2012*

Grey literature

The bibliographical databases mentioned above will not offer an exhaustive collection of all kinds of research or even of published studies (Saini & Shlonsky, 2012). Examples of research that is often not captured include books, reports, master's and doctoral theses and articles published in journals that are not indexed in the databases. Such sources are called *grey literature*. There may also be studies that were never published, either because their scientific quality was not assessed as sufficiently sustainable or due to possible *publication bias*. It has been documented that quantitative primary studies from intervention studies where effect is documented are published more often than studies where effect is not documented (Hopewell et al., 2009). It is, however, uncertain whether a similar publication bias exists in the publication of qualitative studies. Personally, I do not believe that there is an analogous publication bias for qualitative studies.

The search for grey literature takes time and often provides an outcome of limited value. One shortcut may be to consult experts with comprehensive knowledge of the topic, asking if they can provide useful supplements to the search. Even so, some items of grey literature may have insufficient methodological quality to be included, and that may be precisely why they were never published. You should not invest resources to carry out a strategy for this kind of complementary search unless you have good reasons to think it will be worthwhile.

Language

The majority of the research literature in medicine and the health sciences is written in English and therefore is readable by researchers in most high-income countries. Even if you are also literate in other languages like French or German, you may feel a bit odd including articles in less commonly cited languages like Portuguese or Mandarin. Several of the research literature databases do, however, include articles written in languages other than English, often with an abstract in English. It might therefore be possible to assess whether an article written in a language you do not read could still be a potential candidate for inclusion.

For further assessment of the full-text article, we can try digital translation programmes and see how much they help. If an article looks interesting, we can see whether we have or can establish contacts with someone who can help us with a better translation. When identifying a study presenting important findings, we should still maintain a fairly high threshold before we choose to include the article in our analysis. It is very likely that we will not be able to perceive important linguistic nuances of major impact in a qualitative metasynthesis, as with the translation of metaphors, which is a vital step in the analysis process of meta-ethnography (see Chapter 3).

For that matter, we should not imagine that our search strategies will provide access to everything ever written worldwide about a certain topic. No matter how exhaustive a search we conduct, we will always obtain only a selection of the existing research literature. The bibliographic indexing of qualitative studies has many flaws. Depending on the purpose and the available resources, we must make up our minds about how far to proceed regarding articles in languages where our own literacy is limited.

Before you set off seriously

You will need professional assistance to compose and implement the search that will form the basis of your qualitative metasynthesis, independent of any previous experiences and skills in literature search that you or your collaborators may possess. For a qualitative metasynthesis, expert assistance from a research librarian is just as important as statistical support is to a quantitative primary study.

Starting with a couple of test searches based on different combinations of search terms will often be a wise approach. Do not lose courage if your first search generates thousands of hits far from your field of interest, representing little more than garbage. Assessing the number and type of hits will give you some indications of whether you are approaching a feasible task in the next step of screening and reviewing the hits.

It is at least as important to carry out some random checks to find out whether you are on an appropriate track at this point. From such checks, you may adjust your search strategy to make it more precise. New combinations of search terms, operators and other specifications can increase the precision of your final search. At this point, we expect you to have a binding account in which your search strategy is documented, specifying combinations and proper orders in your decision trail for later reports. You may also save your search strategy so that you can update it later if the need arises.

Screening and selection of potentially relevant primary studies

The next step is to organize, screen and select the hits from the literature search. The ultimate purpose is to identify a sample of relevant qualitative primary studies of sufficient methodological quality for upcycling by analysis and synthesis. As in any research project, the character of the sample will have a strong impact on what we can say and how sustainable the evidence will be. That is why we emphasize carrying out this process in a way which can be shared with others, with intersubjectivity and transparency as important and constant reminders.

Reference management

Your efforts to develop an SR will become incoherent and difficult to accomplish unless you use digital software for reference management. My own choice is EndNote, which is well suited for this purpose. When the final literature search is finished, you can import the

literature references from the databases directly to EndNote and combine the files. Do not forget to first document how many hits each of
the search sources provided. Ask the librarian if you need assistance
in this area.

You will notice that several references appear in more than one database, leading to *duplicates* (or triplicates or more) in the combined
file. Duplicates can be deleted in two steps: the first is automatic and
uses an EndNote function, and the second is manual deletion. The latter step is much more time-consuming than the former. However, you
will discover that these efforts are well worth it, as you will be left with
a manageable starting package of unique hits which you subsequently
screen as to relevance and quality. Remember to register the deletion
of duplicates in your decision trail.

Systematic screening and rough classification

In the same way as in most other types of SRs, we follow specific
procedures to identify, select and critically assess potential primary
studies for inclusion in our empirical sample for summing up, analysis and synthesis in qualitative metasynthesis (Dixon-Woods et al.,
2006; Sandelowski & Barroso, 2007; Barnett-Page & Thomas, 2009;
Hannes & Macaitis, 2012; Gough et al., 2017b; Finfgeld-Connett, 2018).
Even when your search has been thoroughly prepared, it will always
include a substantial proportion of references dealing with topics that
are miles away from your actual topic. Such references can be termed
contamination. This phenomenon is a logical consequence of the SR
methodology, in which a fine-toothed comb is often recommended as
the most reliable strategy. This approach is intended to capture all existing research with a systematic and independent review designed to
prevent undesirable skewness by selection of articles.

The described approach resembles the conditions of a *representative sample* used in quantitative studies, rather than a *purposive sample*
commonly used in qualitative studies (Malterud, 2019). For qualitative analysis, I question the commonly expressed aim that the search
should be comprehensive and reproducible (Tong et al., 2012; Booth,
2016) (see Chapter 4). However, the search methodology for SRs appears to have become firmly established and also valid for qualitative
metasyntheses. If we want to comply with this methodological format,
we thus have to follow the core standards underlying these procedures
even as we also take a critical view of the strengths, limitations and
methodological challenges of those principles.

The first step of the review (*screening*) implies weeding out hits that are obvious contamination so that we later can concentrate on references with potential relevance for our research question. Being candidates for inclusion, we can call such articles *candidate articles*. For this categorization to be conducted transparently, we must decide on the criteria to use for inclusion and exclusion, adjust them along the way and register both the criteria and the decision points. At this stage, the procedure deviates from what occurs in an SR of quantitative studies, where inclusion criteria are bindingly decided on in advance (see Chapter 4).

According to the methodological procedures, screening of the literature search hits should be carried out independently and in parallel by at least two researchers. All hits from the literature search are assessed for relevance by each researcher, who highlights references that fulfil the inclusion criteria. The titles of the references are often insufficient to make such an assessment, but the abstract of an article will usually offer the information needed. We then conduct a *conformity check* in which the researchers' assessments are revealed and compared. For some hits, reading the article in full text is necessary to reach a conclusion. Such hits are temporarily included as candidate articles that later become excluded if a closer reading demonstrates that the criteria are not fulfilled.

When the conformity check identifies discrepancies in the researchers' results as to relevance, dialogue and negotiations will usually lead to consensus about inclusion or exclusion. Take care to enter the process and outcomes of such assessments in your decision trail. It is not a goal in itself to include as many primary studies as possible (see Chapter 4) – we want neither too many nor too few. Software has been developed to simplify the screening, comparison and overview of this process, including the provision of specifications for the decision trail regarding reasons for inclusion and exclusion of primary studies.

Reading candidate articles in depth with quality assessment

Following the procedure above, we establish a sample of candidate articles that we retrieve in full text for in-depth reading. First, we conduct another assessment of relevance, which will determine that some of these articles do not actually satisfy our inclusion criteria. We then conduct a *methodological quality assessment* of candidate articles which have passed the relevance test.

Some argue that this kind of quality assessment is unnecessary for qualitative metasyntheses (Carroll et al., 2012), while others note that appropriate criteria can be hard to find (Petticrew, 2015). Dixon-Woods et al. (2007) suggest that it is more important to assess the quality of the results in the primary studies than to assess their methodological procedures, and Sandelowski (2012) uses quality assessment to characterize the included studies but not for exclusion purposes. On this point, I disagree. The candidate articles of a qualitative metasynthesis indeed display great variety in terms of design and theoretical foundation (Saini & Shlonsky, 2012). If the results are to serve as empirical data for our analysis, however, it must be acceptable to insist that these results are the outcome of a process which demonstrates that the basic criteria of research quality have been fulfilled. The overall aim is, after all, the synthesis of existing research evidence.

Others have pointed out that qualitative primary studies often suffer from inadequate accounts concerning methodology (Campbell et al., 2003). To be included in an SR, it is not enough that an article has already been assessed by reviewers and editors before publication.; Assessing the strengths and weaknesses of the empirical data that we use for analysis is vital. There are no good reasons to exempt qualitative studies from methodological quality assessment before inclusion for analysis and synthesis when they serve as incoming evidence for a scientific analysis. In my opinion, methodological quality is a necessary but not sufficient condition for inclusion. Just remember that high scores on the *checklists* do not guarantee that an article will present rich and sustainable results.

Many checklists for methodological assessment of qualitative studies are available (Santiago-Delefosse et al., 2016). Consolidated criteria for reporting qualitative research (*COREQ*) was developed to assess interview studies and focus group studies (Tong et al., 2007). Starting with 22 existing checklists, 76 issues were edited to include 32 questions about research team and reflexivity, study design and data analysis and reporting. Another checklist for qualitative studies developed in the EBM tradition in the series Critical Appraisal Skills Programme (*CASP*) (2013), which was created by an expert group that has piloted and elaborated several versions of the checklist. The 2013 version contains ten questions about aims, appropriateness of qualitative method and research design, recruitment strategy, data collection, researcher-participant relationship, ethical issues, rigorous analysis, statement of findings and value of research. Each question includes some sub-questions for further elaboration.

A third, more comprehensive checklist has been developed by the author of this book (Malterud, 2001b). If you need practice in the methodological appraisal of qualitative studies, this checklist could be useful. You will find detailed questions about study aim, reflexivity, method and design, data collection and sample, theoretical perspectives, analysis, results, discussion, presentation and references. Each question is answered affirmatively, negatively or with a comment. The list is not intended to quantify the methodological quality based on yes-and-no answers. In Fosse's metasynthesis about the role of the NHD at the end of life (2014), this checklist was used for the quality appraisal of candidate articles.

Still, a compound judgment is always necessary when deciding whether an article has sufficient informational power for a certain purpose. It is possible to learn how to execute such judgements, but that takes the experience provided by time and repetition (Thorne, 2017). Even when all methodological rules have been followed assiduously, the results section of a qualitative study may turn out to be weakly or inadequately presented (Eakin & Mykhalovskiy, 2003; Britten et al., 2017). As empirical data for a qualitative metasynthesis, we hope to find primary studies with rich, soundly based and thought-provoking results. Atkins et al. noticed that primary studies with only descriptive findings offer limited useful material, while studies with rich presentations of results based on more comprehensive analysis make more valuable contributions for synthesis (Atkins et al., 2008). Campbell et al. (2003) developed a checklist of 14 themes and 49 questions for the appraisal of incoming evidence, though it has not become widely used.

Popay et al. (1998) recommend that quality appraisal of the results from primary studies emphasize the privileging of lay accounts and subjective meaning, responsiveness to social context and flexible design, theoretical or purposive sampling, adequate description, data quality, theoretical and conceptual adequacy, potential for assessing typicality and – last but not least – relevance to policy. Even when these issues are not specifically included in your checklist, they are useful contributions to an overall appraisal of incoming evidence. When you arrive at analysis and synthesis, you will see their impact more clearly.

Supplementary search

It is almost impossible to work out effective exclusion criteria without losing some primary studies that you would have liked to keep on your list. Still, you may just as well be generous when you use titles and abstracts to exclude a considerable number of the hits initially identified in your search. Keep references when in doubt, but do take care to make notes in your decision trail to be able to transparently sum up your ultimate inclusion criteria (Centre for Reviews and Disssemination, 2008).

This is why we must be prepared for supplementary search, such as screening reference lists in relevant primary studies, review articles or book chapters, or through contact with well-read colleagues

(Atkins et al., 2008; Sandelowski, 2012). This is called *backchaining*. It is also frequently applied in quantitative SRs but is especially important when the topic and method do not easily fit into the bibliographic databases' indexing systems. *Snowball search* is the term for a search strategy in which we follow the threads that we find. For example, an article from the reference list in one article leads to another reference list with several relevant references, and the process repeats. Remember that the more intuitive snowball searches we conduct, the greater the risk of undesirable skewness in the material.

What characterizes your sample?

Before you start to assemble and organize your data as a basis for synthesis, you need to establish a good overview of the primary studies comprising your sample. Knowing the hallmarks of each study and the sample as a whole is crucial to making appropriate interpretations of the data in context. You will also sum up, present and discuss your sample and the impact of its components when you present your metasynthesis as a journal article. With a detailed familiarity with your sample, you are well equipped to create a strategy for extraction and further management of the empirical data from the primary studies.

Flowsheet for search and selection

Your experiences from the test search may rest in your decision trail, while the progression from the literature search itself towards your final selection of included primary studies is displayed in a *flowsheet* that will be included in your published article. A flowsheet template, known as *PRISMA* (Preferred items for systematic reviews and meta-analyses) can be downloaded at http://www.equator-network.org/reporting-guidelines/prisma/.

The literature search in Fosse's metasynthesis about the role of the NHD at the end of life (2014) resulted in 834 hits. Duplicates were deleted, and publications other than journal articles (book chapters, editorials, comments) or using something other than the preferred methodology (quantitative studies) were excluded. The remaining 505 unique hits, all supposed to be reports from qualitative studies, were screened for relevance in title and abstract. During the subsequent screening, all remaining quantitative studies were excluded, as were studies about experiences of health care professionals or studies including only hospitals, hospices or home care services. At the full-text level, 72 candidate articles were assessed for relevance. Ultimately, 14 qualitative primary studies were included for analysis and synthesis (see Figure 2.1).

PRISMA 2009 Flow Diagram

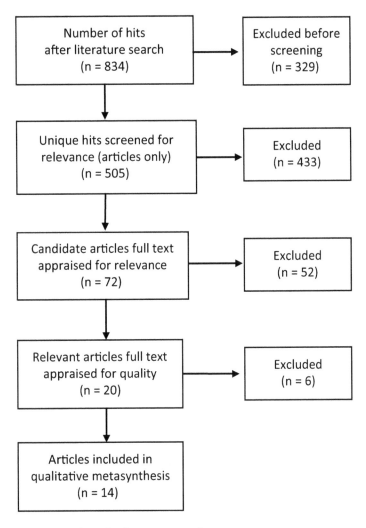

Figure 2.1 Flowsheet for literature search.

Source: Adapted from (Fosse et al., 2014). PRISMA 2009 Flow Diagram, Moher D, Liberati A, Tetzlaff J, Altman DG, The PRISMA Group (2009). Preferred Reporting Items for Systematic Reviews and Meta-Analyses: The PRISMA Statement. PLoS Med 6(6): e1000097. doi:10.1371/journal.pmed1000097

Hallmarks of the primary studies

When the selection process is concluded, you can establish a table in which you systematize the hallmarks of each primary study included. The table should contain columns for first author, year of publication, country, title, design and data collection, context and relevant characteristics of the study population (such as number, age, gender and duration of illness). This table may be compared to an overview of relevant demographic data for the participants in a focus group study, but here the units to be mapped and organized are the primary studies themselves. Table 2.1 demonstrates how Fosse et al. (2014) carried out this step. Their study included data from a total of 70 patients and 312 family members based on 10 studies with individual interviews, 3 focus group studies and a survey with open-ended answers. Similarly, Dahl et al., in their meta-ethnography about lesbian families encountering the maternity ward (2013), included data from 13 primary studies with a total of 242 participants (biological mothers, co-mothers, nurses) from 5 countries. At this stage of the process, you may prefer to work with full-text printouts of the articles – it is useful to become acquainted with the visual expressions of each article and to develop a sense of how the different authors express themselves.

You will probably soon notice that many of the articles are not especially similar. It is a challenge to find good terms to classify hallmarks across articles, but you should not invest too much effort in coordinating methodological terminology across studies. There are innumerable ways to categorize qualitative studies (Creswell, 2013), and you cannot expect that "your" authors will all speak the same language in this regard. A pragmatic, intermediate solution is to register expressions and terms as they are presented in each article. Later, when you have completed a thorough reading of all the primary studies, you can consider whether you have the basis for a more consistent presentation of similarities and differences in their design and methodology.

Preparing an SR based on quantitative data, it may be practical to combine the overview of articles with data extraction, establishing columns for major findings and the strengths and weaknesses of the studies in the table. With qualitative metasynthesis, my recommendation is to separate the process of organizing the overview of studies' hallmarks from the process of data extraction, in which you identify and organize the results from the primary studies. It may be tempting to try to incorporate everything. Assume that you at this step first and foremost develop a key map which simplifies your overview of the sample during the subsequent work. Later, you will organize the data extraction overview.

Table 2.1 Overview of included studies.

FIRST AUTHOR YEAR	LAND	TITLE	DATA COLLECTION	CONTEXT	PARTICIPANTS
Caron (2005)	Canada	End-of-life decision-making in dementia: the perspective of family caregivers	In-depth interviews, open-ended questions	University geriatric institute and publicly funded long-term care centre	24 family members
Dreyer (2009)	Norway	Autonomy at the end of life: life-prolonging treatment in nursing homes – relatives' role in the decision-making process	Semi-structured in-depth interviews	Nursing homes from various geographical and demographic areas in Norway	15 family members
Franklin (2006)	Sweden	Views on dignity of elderly nursing home residents	Semi-structured in-depth interviews	Nursing home patients in Sweden	12 patients
Lambert (2005)	Canada	Factors affecting long-term-care residents' decision-making process as they formulate advance directives	Semi-structured in-depth interview	Semi-privately funded not-for-profit nursing home in Ontario	9 patients
Lopez (2009)	USA	Doing what's best: decisions by families of acutely ill nursing home residents	In-depth interview, open-ended questions	Four nursing homes in Massachusetts	12 family members

(Continued)

FIRST AUTHOR YEAR	LAND	TITLE	DATA COLLECTION	CONTEXT	PARTICIPANTS
Munn (2008)	USA	The end-of-life experience in long-term care: five themes identified from focus groups with residents, family members, and staff	Focus groups	Five nursing homes and eight residential-care and assisted-living facilities in North Carolina	11 patients, 19 family members, 35 staff
Ott (2008)	USA	Views of African American nursing home residents about living wills	Focus groups	African-Americans from three not-for-profit nursing homes in a metropolitan area in the northeastern United States	28 patients
Shield (2005)	USA	Physicians "missing in action": family perspectives on physician and staff problems in end-of-life care in nursing homes	In-depth semi-structured telephone interview	A subsample of quantitative survey respondents regarding bereaved family members' perceptions of end-of-life care	54 family members[a]
Teno (2001)	USA	Patient-focused, family-centred end-of-life medical care: views of the guidelines and bereaved family members	Focus groups	Nursing homes, hospices and hospitals in Arizona, Massachusetts, New York	42 family members

(Continued)

Author (year)	Country	Title	Method	Sample	N
Towsley (2011)	USA	Mixed messages: nursing home resident preferences about care at end of life	Semi-structured in-depth interviews	Cognitively able residents from two urban nursing homes	10 patients
Vohra (2006)	Canada	The last word: family members' descriptions of end-of-life care in long-term care facilities	Open-ended question in postal survey	Various long-term care facilities in south-central Ontario	104 family members
Waldrop (2012)	USA	The living-dying interval in nursing home-based end-of-life care: family caregivers' experiences	In-depth interviews, open-ended questions	Nursing homes in northeastern New York state	31 family members
Wetle (2005)	USA	Family perspectives on end-of-life care experiences in nursing homes	In-depth semi-structured telephone interviews	A subsample of quantitative survey respondents regarding bereaved family members' perceptions of end-of-life care	54 family members[a]
Wilson (1999)	USA	Family perspectives on dying in long-term care settings	Semi-structured in-depth interviews	11 long-term care facilities in a large city in the Midwestern United States: family members with a loss within the past four weeks	11 family members

Source: Fosse et al., 2014.
a Same subsample.

Identification of results from the primary studies

Data extraction is the process by which we single out and collect relevant information from the included studies. During analysis and synthesis, you continue to work with empirical data – the results that you have systematically identified and marked in the articles in your sample. The results in the primary studies are your point of departure for upcycling, not their authors' conclusions or comments on what others have written about analogous topics. Therefore, it would be plausible to expect that you would find what you are looking for in the results section of an article. You could consider starting with the results as presented by the abstract of the article, followed by their elaboration in the results section.

This is, however, a part of the process about which you will not find extensive descriptions in the methodology literature and which contains many challenges. Unfortunately, you will probably realize that several of the articles which you previously accepted regarding methodology still do not offer much in the way of substantive results (Thorne, 2017). Campbell et al. describe data extraction as a time-consuming and challenging stage of analysis, since primary studies often present their results vaguely and incompletely (Campbell et al., 2003). Sometimes you will find results sections that are barely distinguishable from the preconceptions presented in the introduction. In other cases, you may read results from a descriptive study that appear rather trivial where substantive contributions are limited (Sandelowski, 2012).

Some authors include many references to previous research in the results section, most often to compare their own findings and discuss differences and similarities. In such cases, it may be necessary to read very meticulously to clarify which segments of the text actually represent the findings of the article and its author(s). In some articles, the findings are elaborated and extended in the discussion paragraphs of the article, often in a more detailed way that may contribute to increased information power. In still other articles the conclusion will present the main findings most clearly. You will probably also encounter articles in which the results section contains little analytic text and an abundance of quotations. Sandelowsky (2012) emphasizes that we must distinguish between results arising out of researcher interpretations from the data that legitimize or illustrate these interpretations, such as coding schemes, field notes and quotations. In any case, I expect you to be surprised and a bit disappointed when you discover how many articles present results with limited sustainability (Britten et al., 2017).

Personally, I usually apply a text marker when I first read a primary study closely. I highlight everything I consider to be results which will constitute the core of texts that will proceed to analysis after data extraction. To start with, I also incorporate some quotations that adequately illustrate the results, while I leave quotations that appear more disconnected to the side. I am reluctant to classify text passages with several references as results. You should therefore be selective but also a little generous. You will become very familiar with these text passages, and, little by little, you will be able to recognize empirical data with appropriate *information power* (Malterud et al., 2016b).

This part of the process may be compared to the identification of meaning units in a thematic cross-case analysis in a qualitative primary study (Malterud, 2012). In that context, too, we do not expect every part of the transcript to contribute information about what we want to explore. In qualitative metasynthesis, we set off in pursuit of the actual authorial contribution to the existing knowledge about our research question.

Data extraction from qualitative studies implies subjective and systematic interpretations. Repeatability and independence, which are important criteria for this stage in other SRs, become irrelevant and even misleading (see Chapter 4). Intersubjectivity must be taken care of in other ways than having another researcher select exactly the same text segments that you did. You owe your reader sufficient visibility into your process to understand the important choices you have made. Still, it is always useful to collaborate with at least one person during this process and engage in a continual dialogue about what will be brought along further on and why those decisions are made. If your team is too large, however, you can expect finicky and time-consuming negotiations that do not always benefit the process.

Use your decision trail to register challenges, dilemmas and choices, but never let the technical details and their challenges in this first part of the research process overshadow your goal. Interpretation and synthesis is what all these data are supposed to serve (Popay et al., 1998; Thorne, 2015; Britten et al., 2017; Thorne, 2017). You can easily get lost in literature accumulation and management. If so, time and resources may be spent before you arrive at analysis and synthesis, the major interpretative pivot point of this research method.

Organizing the material from data extraction

Taste, temper and practicalities will influence how you choose to organize the material that you have identified. For quantitative primary studies, a template may help you develop a diagram for data extraction, while in qualitative metasynthesis, the procedure will usually be different.

I prefer to use full-text printouts for identifying the text segments that communicate results from the primary studies. During my thorough reading of the articles, I have already highlighted such text segments with a marker. These text selections are my most important empirical data for further analysis and synthesis. Along your way, you will also often want to read these segments in the contexts where their authors originally presented them, and full-text printouts with highlighted results are a convenient way to achieve that goal. The more articles you have included, the more challenging it will be to preserve an overview.

I do not use any specific software for qualitative analysis in this process. I prefer to establish a flexible matrix as my tool for organizing these text segments, whether my choice will be to proceed along a digital or analogue path later on. In the CFS/ME metasynthesis, we inserted sticky notes onto a large sheet of paper, with the full-text printouts easily available and sorted alphabetically (Larun & Malterud, 2007). Digital tools may, however, be more effective and flexible than loose slips of paper. In the metasynthesis about obesity and stigma in the health care system, the selected text segments were entered verbatim into columns in an MS Excel spreadsheet (Malterud & Ulriksen, 2011). The way one organizes the matrix is an essential part of the analysis (see Chapter 3). Before we go through the specific procedures, we can first take a step back to study some principles of qualitative metasynthesis which can be complied with while taking into account different analytic strategies and levels of ambition.

3   Analysis and synthesis

Interpretation of the results from the primary studies

A systematic literature review that sums up existing research is the starting point for qualitative metasynthesis. When you have identified and organized the primary studies you want to include and have retrieved sustainable results text sections from them, you are ready to set out on analysis and synthesis. Several procedures have been developed for this purpose, but we first examine certain basic, generic principles. This chapter offers a detailed presentation of the procedure, illustrated by a practical example in which meta-ethnography has been applied.

Synthesis is more than summary and renarration

In qualitative metasynthesis, we upcycle existing knowledge, using analysis where synthesis is supposed to lead us towards something different and more than the sum of the parts (Riese et al., 2014). Thorne et al. (2004) emphasize that metasynthesis is something other than simply organizing and presenting empirical data:

> We understand that product to be fundamentally different from the original parts, capable of substantiating a more convincing argument about the major theoretical elements within the phenomenon of interest and positioned to advance the science in that particular substantive field more forcefully.

Secondary analysis, in which qualitative data developed for a certain purpose are reanalysed for another purpose, is not the same as metasynthesis (Dixon-Woods et al., 2005). Interview data originally collected to study symptom experiences might for example also contain interesting data about health care encounters. In such cases, the original data could be reused to conduct a secondary analysis, writing a new article in which the secondary analysis is used to explore the new aim. In metasynthesis, the results from the primary studies – not the original raw data underlying those results – constitute the point of departure for analysis and synthesis.

You start by assessing whether the data are sufficiently sustainable to be upcycled in a systematic analysis. Your material should be neither too vast, which will endanger your ability to maintain an overview, nor too meagre, in which case you will lack enough building blocks. If only three qualitative studies remain on your list after your review and screening, it is probably better to moderate your ambitions and sum them up in a narrative review rather than struggling to present a more comprehensive course of action. If, on the other hand, you have ample material, such as ten primary studies featuring powerful presentations of results, you can use your results as data for a proper metasynthesis.

It is a great advantage if you have previously conducted analysis of qualitative data in an empirical primary study before you set out on a qualitative metasynthesis. You will notice that many steps are analogous, but something is different. Analysis and synthesis are conducted according to the same criteria of critical, systematic reflection as in any qualitative analysis. Several strategies for analysis are available (Dixon-Woods et al., 2005; Bondas & Hall, 2007b; Barnett-Page & Thomas, 2009; Hannes & Macaitis, 2012; Finfgeld-Connett, 2018). Some researchers choose to conduct a thematic analysis as in a primary study with empirical data, while exhibiting different levels of theoretical commitment (Braun & Clarke, 2006; Thorne, 2008; Malterud, 2012). Others use a methodology especially developed for qualitative metasynthesis. In her study about the role of the nursing home doctor (NHD) at the end of life, Fosse decided, after consulting her supervisors and collaborators, to use meta-ethnography, a method that has been thoroughly described and frequently used (Noblit & Hare, 1988). See below for more about meta-ethnography.

Levels of interpretation – concepts of first, second and third orders

In a qualitative empirical primary study, we employ several levels of interpretation. The point of departure could be an event leading to certain experiences on which the participant elaborates and reports in some form of dialogue with the researcher. What will be told is filtered by the participant's judgments and memories and by the attentiveness of the researcher. This version of the story is assembled in a material format like an audio recording and a transcription thereof. When the researcher uses the transcript as data for analysis, the event has already been interpreted at several stages.

The analysis is the most explicit level of interpretation. Here, the researcher, supported by relevant theoretical perspectives, reads, interprets and reflects upon the data so that the interpretation leads to new knowledge (Malterud, 2016). Reflexivity implies among other things that we continuously make up our minds regarding the level of interpretation we are using. With metasynthesis, this often leads to challenges, since we will handle new levels of interpretation without having thorough knowledge about the interpretations already reported in the primary study.

The sociologist and philosopher Alfred Schütz belonged to the phenomenological tradition. He presented a terminology (1962) that distinguishes between concepts of first and second order, depending on the level of analytic ambition. *First-order concepts* are made up by individuals' understandings in everyday language, for our purpose expressed as empirical raw data in statements from participants in focus groups or individual interviews. In a descriptive study, where participant accounts are summed up with very limited theoretical commitment, the terms used in the results section may also be considered first-order concepts. It is, however, not always easy to distinguish levels (Atkins et al., 2008). *Second-order concepts* evolve from the systematic interpretations, for our purpose made by the researcher of the participants' first-order statements, preferably supported by a theoretical frame of reference. The results from a qualitative primary study of proper quality are closer to second- than first-order concepts.

Britten et al. (2002) apply these concepts in their meta-ethnography about the lay meanings of medicines. Initially, the authors organize the main findings from the primary studies thematically. According to the authors, if only limited interpretation has taken place through this sorting, what ensues remain second-order concepts. Afterwards, a synthesis leading towards *third-order concepts* is conducted. Saini and Shlonsky (2012) apply a similar terminology. The vocabulary exercised in the methodological literature about metasynthesis is, however, not consistent. First, second and third orders are used to denote both concepts and levels of analysis (Fisher et al., 2006; Atkins et al., 2008; Malpass et al., 2009; Murray et al., 2015). The most important point, therefore, is that we have sufficient insight to express what we have done in a comprehensible and consequential way that contributes to intersubjectivity.

In qualitative metasynthesis, we can simplify these matters by stating that raw data may be equated with first-order concepts, the results from primary studies with second-order concepts and the endpoints of the metasynthesis as third-order concepts. The condition for this claim is that we accomplish an interpretative synthesis in which the results from existing research are elaborated and expanded upon, as opposed to a descriptive systematic review (SR) that merely sums up and repeats existing knowledge (Walsh & Downe, 2005; Saini & Shlonsky, 2012; Thorne, 2015).

Different strategies for metasynthesis

Metasynthesis, as applied in this book, is a method approaching not only the content but also the meaning of the results from the primary studies included for analysis. Paterson et al. (2001) use the term *metastudy* as an overarching concept that includes, besides metasynthesis, two additional possible review types, emphasizing theoretical perspectives or methodological strategies, respectively. They call the latter *meta-methodical studies.* The aim of this kind of study is to explore and evaluate the use and impact of the methodological presuppositions in primary studies and metasyntheses and evaluate their consequences for management and interpretation.

Meta-methodical studies that emphasize methods in qualitative metasynthesis can also provide useful contributions that suggest approaches to be chosen for further research into a given topic. Paterson et al. (2001) describe, for example, how the evolution of methodology in qualitative studies about chronic disease developed to better accommodate the pain, fatigue and social distance experienced by patients with terminal cancer. In this book, we will not discuss in great depth the procedures used in meta-methodical studies, but we will apply certain results and conclusions to deepen our insights into some methodological concerns at play in qualitative primary studies and metasyntheses. The classification of different qualitative methodological approaches involves, however, many challenges, and this is true of not only primary studies (Kastner et al., 2012).

Bondas and Hall (2007b) reviewed 45 qualitative health sciences metasyntheses published between 1994 and 2006 and observed that more than half reported using the meta-ethnography method (Noblit & Hare, 1988). In several other metasyntheses, modified versions of meta-ethnography were used, with or without explicit reference. Similarly, Dixon-Woods et al. (2007) reviewed 42 qualitative syntheses of qualitative research in health and health care published between 1988 and 2004. Here, too, meta-ethnography was the most frequently used method, often with adaptations. Hannes and Macaitis (2012) and France et al. (2014) have also confirmed this trend.

Several metasyntheses examined in these meta-methodical studies were conducted using well-known generic methods for analysis in qualitative primary studies, such as grounded theory, hermeneutic-phenomenological analysis, cross-case analysis, content analysis or Paul Ricoeur's text analysis. Some authors presented their methods with reference to previous studies conducted by others, while others used their own methods for analysis (Paterson et al., 2001).

In all the meta-methodical studies presented above, the authors point out that the metasynthesis method is often insufficiently described in the articles, or that adequate agreement between the method described and the actual presentation in the article is lacking. They also call for further information about the search strategies used. From these findings, we have good reason to ask whether the basic criteria for an SR have been met. There are, however, indications that these issues have improved to some extent in recent years (Hannes & Macaitis, 2012).

In addition to the meta-methodical studies, a lot of review articles and book chapters present and discuss various analytical methods for metasynthesis (Dixon-Woods et al., 2005; Mays et al., 2005; Bondas & Hall, 2007a; Barnett-Page & Thomas, 2009; Sandelowski, 2012; Gough et al., 2017b; Finfgeld-Connett, 2018). Here, we also find suggestions to employ the traditional methods of analysis used in qualitative primary studies, such as grounded theory, cross-case thematic analysis, framework analysis or content analysis. Bayesian analysis is mentioned in several of the articles in connection with mixed-method studies (Spiegelhalter et al., 2000). This is, however, a specific strategy for the statistical calculation of probability that has limited relevance for qualitative metasynthesis.

Apart from meta-ethnography (Noblit & Hare, 1988), some methods have also been specifically developed for qualitative metasynthesis. Among them, the most frequently used appear to be *critical interpretive synthesis* (Dixon-Woods et al., 2006), *thematic synthesis* (Thomas & Harden, 2008) and *realist synthesis* (Wong et al., 2013). Below you will find a detailed presentation of the major principles and procedures for meta-ethnography, followed by brief accounts of critical interpretative synthesis, thematic synthesis and realist synthesis.

Meta-ethnography

Meta-ethnography is the method which established the point of departure for qualitative metasynthesis and still remains its most commonly used approach. The method was presented with a detailed description of principles, procedures and concepts, along with an emphasis on certain fundamental principles from the philosophy of science.

If we want to refer to and use this method, it is essential to learn the tools of the trade and know what distinguishes it from related methods for synthesis. It will also be necessary to understand how it can be accomplished in practice.

Background

George W. Noblit and R. Dwight Hare, ethnographers in education research, were the first to develop and present a specific method for the synthesis of qualitative studies (1988). The authors were social scientists with a special interest in how knowledge from qualitative studies could help explain social and cultural phenomena. Noblit and Hare argued that all synthesis is interpretation, no matter whether it is accomplished with qualitative or quantitative research methods. By juxtaposing several existing studies, the researcher infuses meaning into what s/he sees, in the same way that ethnographers interpret their observations while positioned in a certain culture. For synthesis, Noblit and Hare used ethnographic primary studies from education research, based on long-lasting and intensive observation, interaction and review of documents. Still, they do not restrict the method exclusively to ethnographic studies or principles.

Noblit and Hare emphasize that meta-ethnography is an inductive method belonging to the interpretative paradigm, that its synthesis implies interpretation rather than merely description and that context is an essential precondition for understanding (Noblit & Hare, 1988). The authors offer a procedure with seven steps that constitute a systematic approach that is possible to follow, explain and discuss.

Metaphors and translations

The heart of the matter in meta-ethnography is to take a stand as to how the main findings of the primary studies included relate to one another in the ways they have been interpreted and presented by their authors (France et al., 2014). An intuitive review is not as simple, because each study's findings are usually very heterogeneously expressed due to different methodological traditions and theoretical perspectives.

In everyday speech, *metaphor* is "a figure of speech in which a word or phrase literally denoting one kind of object or idea is used in place of another to suggest a likeness or analogy between them" (Merriam Webster Dictionary). In their book about meta-ethnography, Noblit and Hare (1988) apply the metaphor concept to the main expressions and notions used by the primary study authors in sharing their findings. At an early stage of our review of the empirical data, we will identify these kinds of text segments, which are those with sufficient capacity and strength to incorporate the main ethnographic findings. Noblit and Hare call this *metaphoric reduction.*

Translation is the term used by Noblit and Hare for the subsequent process of comparing relevant metaphors from the primary studies included (Noblit & Hare, 1988). The theoretical arguments for this concept and mode of thought build on the work of the sociologist Stephen P. Turner (1980), who insists that all explanations are based on comparisons achieved by means of translation. Noblit and Hare clarify that synthesis in meta-ethnography involves translating qualitative studies into one another by using the metaphors employed in the results they report. The translation is *idiomatic*, focusing on the meaning content rather than on literal equivalents (Noblit & Hare, 1988). Consequently, we are not discussing the direct translation referred to in everyday speech but to a systematic exploration of similarities and differences between the expressions used by the various authors to present their results.

Synthesis implies the transformation of concepts dealing with related issues into an overarching third-order concept. Noblit and Hare insist that the researcher must be multilingual (in a metaphorical sense), with the capacity to compare nuances of similarities and differences in order to accommodate the distinctive character of each study. They remind us that such translations always are imprinted by the frames of reference and preconceptions of the researcher.

Analytical perspectives

Noblit and Hare recommend that, early in the process, we decide on a primary perspective of either *reciprocal translation analysis*, in which we mutually translate different concepts for related phenomena into one another, or *refutational synthesis*, in which contrasts and contradictions in the material are emphasized.

Subsequently, we can also use the analysis to develop a *lines-of-argument synthesis* in which we present our synthesis as a logical connection between the main findings from the previous analytical strategies. This perspective on analysis requires rich and sustainable data with proper informational power. Before setting out, we must decide whether or not the empirical foundation is sufficient, as it turned out to be in the metasynthesis about experiences with Chronic fatigue syndrome/ Myalgic encephalopathy (CFS/ME) (Larun & Malterud, 2007).

Strategy for analysis – seven steps

Noblit & Hare (1988) presented their strategy for analysis in seven steps. Since 1988, however, the possibilities of advanced literature searches have exploded and the methodologies of qualitative research as well as SRs have been extensively elaborated. The specific conduct of the research process will therefore take a somewhat different course today than when meta-ethnography was first developed. Still, it is not difficult to follow the original understanding of the seven steps, although the passage between the steps will likely be more fluid in practice. How our practical procedures are positioned according to these steps is thus a matter for discussion, and we choose to regard these steps as recommendations. Table 3.1 presents the analytical steps with my elaborations, which we can describe, using Noblit and Hare's own terminology, as translations into contemporary research realities.

The first three steps prior to analysis and synthesis have already been detailed in Chapters 1 and 2. Below, we render concrete the moves needed for the specific conduct of analysis and synthesis in steps 4–6, supported by Noblit and Hare's terminology and theoretical frame of reference (Noblit & Hare, 1988). The last step – communication and writing – is dealt with in the final paragraph of this chapter.

The matrix as a tool for analysis

Even when you have a sample of manageable size, it can be challenging to maintain an overview of the empirical material, which is comprised of the selected text segments that you have identified during data extraction (see previous chapter). It is therefore a good idea to start the analysis by refreshing your familiarity with each primary study. When you develop your synthesis in the next phase by identifying, comparing and translating relevant metaphors for each study, it is also useful to have an idea about which main themes from your material can shed light on your aim. This may be compared with step 1 in systematic text condensation, a method for thematic cross-case analysis of qualitative data (Malterud, 2012).

During data extraction, you will have complied with Noblit and Hare's recommendations to concentrate on text segments containing words and expressions – metaphors – that transmit the authors' core concepts regarding their major findings. The rest you have let lie. You will, however, notice that the extent of text being extracted here is much smaller than in a qualitative primary study. Therefore, it is all the better when the texts contain sustainable and upcyclable expressions of the main findings.

Table 3.1 Overview of the seven steps of meta-ethnography.

Step	Noblit and Hare	My elaboration – management in practice
1	Getting started	Articulate aim and search strategy, write protocol, conduct literature search.
2	Deciding what is relevant to the initial interest	Review literature search, develop criteria for inclusion, exclude duplicates and hits whose titles or abstracts do not comply with criteria, appraise the full text of candidate studies, establish sample of primary studies included, prepare an outline of those studies.
3	Reading the studies	Thorough reading of the full text of the primary studies included to localize the results from the primary studies, which constitute the empirical material for metasynthesis, and to obtain an overview of themes and metaphors.
4	Determining how the studies are related	Data extraction, in which the empirical data are organized in a matrix with relevant themes and metaphors for each primary study listed in vertical columns, starting with a rich index study.
5	Translating the studies into one another	Systematic examination and organization of text segments with results having related themes and metaphors across studies in the horizontal rows in the matrix, emphasizing similarities and differences in expressions.
6	Synthesizing translations	Review of each horizontal row to develop an overarching translation which embraces all themes and metaphors expressed as a new concept that offers an original and independent understanding of the findings.
7	Expressing the synthesis	Elaborate and give the grounds for the meaning content in the expressions from the synthesis mediated by the new translation, write the results paragraphs for the metasynthesis article.

Source: After (Noblit & Hare, 1988).

Take your time in the initial moves of analysis to organize your data before you set out on the synthesis proper. The *matrix* is used as a tool to cut and paste and move the text segments with metaphors and results from cell to cell. First, you establish the matrix, assigning a column to each primary study and entering the first author and year of publication for each study in the upper row. Do not forget to include year of publication, since the same author or different authors with identical last names could have contributed several different primary studies among those you have included.

Subsequently, you systematically enter or paste the selected text segments from each primary study into the column assigned to the actual primary study. The sequence of text segments is determined by continuous assessments of which text segments are related across studies, so that the rows in the matrix finally contain data and metaphors with notable common features while simultaneously making differences and contrasts visible. The first sequences of these efforts might well be carried out by the joint research team, who can discuss and negotiate about which text segments are related and into which cells they should thus be entered (Thorne, 2017). By following this approach, you are systematically deciding how the studies are related and whether the results are sustainable while preparing for the next step of analysis, in which you translate the metaphors into one another.

It is essential to establish a working method that enables you to operate flexibly and inductively, in which the location of every text segment is adjusted as you decide on what is related to it, both in each primary study and across the totality of them. In a digital spreadsheet, it is easy to move content from cell to cell and try out different patterns of related data. You can apply similar principles if you choose to work with sticky notes.

If you use a spreadsheet for your matrix, you save it with a new name indicating date and time after every session. In Fosse's metasynthesis about the role of the NHD at the end of life (2014), five versions of the matrix were saved as the process of analysis and synthesis unfolded. If you work on paper, you can take photos of the matrix at different stages. In this way, it is easy to create space for reflection, return to previous steps and adjust the course when appropriate.

A specific example of analysis and synthesis

Table 3.2 presents an excerpt of a matrix for a meta-ethnography of qualitative studies about stigma and obesity in health care (Malterud & Ulriksen, 2011). In presenting the process of analysis, I chose this study as an example instead of Fosse's study because this illustration of the matrix was included in the published article. Remember that this is only a highly simplified snapshot of an inductive and iterative process of systematic interpretation that was far more dynamic and complex than the illustration makes it appear. The matrix is a flexible document in which the distribution of text segments in the different cells reflects patterns of associations between related cell contents that have been organized and reorganized several times. Metaphors, indicating substantial expressions and concepts in the text segments of primary study results, appear in bold text.

Table 3.2 Simplified excerpt of matrix for synthesis and analysis with metaphors in bold.

Brown 2006	Rogge 2004	Merrill 2008	Wright 1998	Brown 2007	Thomas 2008	Reed 2003	Díaz 2007	Epstein 2005	Our translation	STIGMA PATTERN
(1) Your weight is a **problem** (2) **Minimal support** was offered along with practical advice	It **oughta be easy** to lose 20 pounds before the operation	Well, you **just have to stop** eating	Fat is unhealthy and poses serious risks, **go home and lose weight** before surgery			**Just drink more water** and push yourself away from the table			**Well, you just have to stop eating**	Apparently proper advice, probably well intended – yet perceived as **patronizing**
(1) Strong sense of **personal responsibility**, (2) Imagine the **worst must be thought about** them	(1) Obese people agree with the construction of obesity as **their own fault** (2) Assume obesity is due to **overindulgence** and eating out (3) The doctor will not be thrilled to hear that I have gained weight	**Persistence of trying** to control or lose weight		The importance of **personal lifestyles**	All participants **had attempted** to lose weight numerous times in their lives		**Familiarity with weight loss methods** and failed weight loss attempts	(1) A problem that had been caused and should **be managed by the patients** themselves, (2) Patients can be in **denial**, reluctant to accept responsibility, want the doctor to take ownership	**The personal responsibility of obesity**	
They're **putting everything down to your weight**		Having their **weight addressed** instead of the health problem							**Attributing any problem to body weight**	

Source: After (Malterud & Ulriksen, 2011).

At an early stage of this meta-ethnography, we appraised our data and found them sufficiently sustainable to undertake a reciprocal translation analysis. Initially, we therefore emphasized similarities between metaphors and results from the different primary studies. We identified an *index study* – a primary study that stood out by presenting especially rich and sustainable results when compared to the other included studies (Brown et al., 2006). Another option is to choose the oldest primary study as your index study (Campbell et al., 2003).

We assigned the outer left column to the index study and entered relevant short segments of texts from the results, including and highlighting the metaphors, in the cells in that column. Then we carried out a similar systematic reading of the next primary study (Rogge et al., 2004), positioning results text segments with metaphors and meanings related to the index study in cells in the appropriate row. This procedure implies metaphoric reduction of second-order concepts (see above). Sometimes, however, the actual primary study is more of a descriptive repetition of the participants' stories, without much theoretical support. In such cases, this course of action will mean a metaphoric reduction of first-order concepts. We will, however, not get overly caught up in these classifications here. Instead, we will establish an ambition that our analysis will lead to synthesis of a higher order than found in the primary studies. When using spreadsheets in this process, it can be smart to zoom in and out, depending on whether you looking for an overview or for details at a given moment. You should certainly take some time to establish an appropriate font size and formatting for the cells. It is important that you are able to observe all text in each cell (use the wrap text function) while retaining a bird's-eye perspective.

When all the identified results from every primary study included had been organized in a similar fashion, we had established the draft of a map exhibiting our initial analysis of how the studies were related. This map also demonstrated visually which primary studies could contribute with significant data to the analysis and which offered more limited accounts. During this process, we also noticed some important nuances in some of the more limited primary studies. A systematic appraisal of such issues can be compared to *sensitivity analysis* in quantitative meta-analysis, where the researcher calculates how the result is influenced by variations or changes in the primary studies that serve as the basis for analysis (Cochrane Collaboration, 2011). For a qualitative metasynthesis, the most important element is to reflect upon how we will emphasize different parts of the empirical material.

Our metasynthesis about obesity and stigma in health care was supported by Foucault's theoretical perspectives (1988) (pp. 16–63) about symbolic power and discursive practices. Keeping these ideas in mind and considering how the metaphors we had identified could best elucidate our aim, we established three main themes. We focused consecutively on attitudes related to (1) patronizing, (2) exclusion and (3) contempt. All the primary studies contributed, although to different degrees, to all three themes. Setting out by organizing the data in these main themes should not be mistaken for a traditional thematic analysis. This is only a point of departure for the process of analysis proper, leading to synthesis. Subsequently, we carried out complete meta-ethnographic syntheses with metaphoric reductions and translations for each one of the three themes.

During the process, the themes, rows and our understanding of how text segments and metaphors are related will be adjusted several times. Therefore, we need tools that are flexible and offer an outline adequate for accomplishing an interpretative, inductive analysis. Saving different versions of the matrix along the way will enable you to share the path you have followed. These procedures will also be of help when you decide to take a step backwards to adjust your direction. The way I present the process here could be perceived as analogous to standard methods for cross-case analysis of qualitative primary data with different levels of theoretical commitment (Malterud, 2012; Miles et al., 2014). However, meta-ethnography is distinguished by an overall mission of translating metaphors that is expected to be clearly expressed in process and presentation. This is the step in which the synthesis itself is accomplished.

We review systematically each of the horizontal rows to establish an overarching translation with a new expression that covers all vital evidence and metaphors and provides an original and independent understanding of the findings. In the example, we have exhibited translations and synthesis in the two columns to the right, here presented as three aspects of the theme of being patronizing. Please note that our translation for one such aspect is nearly identical to text found in one of the primary studies. While Noblit & Hare (1988) recommend putting significant effort into developing our own translations, we will sometimes accept that one of the authors have provided a metaphor that incorporates the translation across relevant studies better that we could have done it ourselves. In the column on the far right, we have taken our three translations as our point of departure and amalgamated them as third-order concepts. Please note that this is not the final synthesis or result – rather, it is a cue containing the major aspects of the analysis that will subsequently be spelled out. Presenting the results of any synthesis will require much more than five or six words.

We carried out similar translations for the other two main themes. We then undertook a refutational synthesis for all three main themes, seeking contradictions in our data. This stage provides important points of reference for the final synthesis, where we lean towards the theoretical perspectives we have prioritized, together with an overall exploration of the data that serve as the basis of the translations. We presented the synthesis in the form of a line-of-argument synthesis. We put significant effort into finding expressions with the best capacity to recontextualize and integrate what we have processed, while at the same time revealing something new and relevant. This was how we approached one of the three dimensions of stigma and obesity in health care presented in the article (Malterud & Ulriksen, 2011). Analysis and synthesis were accomplished in a similar way in Fosse's project (2014).

Contemporary meta-ethnography

Meta-ethnography was introduced at a time when qualitative research methods were still neither very widespread nor broadly recognized. Ethnographic methodology is rooted in social anthropology and refers to theories about culture, society and symbols (Malinowski, 1944; Garfinkel, 1967; Atkinson & Hammersley, 1994). Ethnographic analysis is often based on fieldwork with participant observation (Maanen, 2011). Such strategies have been used for social science research in different disciplines, including by educational researchers like Noblit and Hare. Today, some researchers have legitimate reservations about the concept of ethnography used in this context (Dixon-Woods et al., 2006; Major & Savin-Baden, 2010). For metasyntheses of medical and health research, it might be more constructive to bring along the major principles presented by Noblit and Hare rather than arguing that this is supposed to be ethnography in the contemporary meaning of the term.

The method was also established long before bibliographic research databases and digital tools for literature searches were made available. Noblit and Hare's specification of procedures do not include what we now consider to be methodological tools for the data collection in an SR (see Chapter 2). To be sure, there are examples showing that meta-ethnography can be used for the synthesis of primary studies selected in a different way than by a systematic search, such as a synthesis of primary studies that all arise from the same research project (Steihaug et al., 2016). It is especially important in such cases to make explicit the premises underlying the sample and to discuss their impact.

Noblit and Hare (1988) illustrate the practical accomplishment of meta-ethnography by referring to a synthesis based on two to four in-depth ethnographic studies. Today, even with a sharply focused aim and a critical review of the literature search as to relevance and quality, you will usually end up with a much larger sample of primary studies included. In a meta-methodical study, France et al. (2014) identified 32 meta-ethnographies about health or health care published in 2012 or 2013, based on syntheses of 3 to 77 primary studies, with a median of 18. They suggest that the trend is towards ever-increasing sample sizes, leading to reflections about what number is useful or even necessary. A manageable sample of primary studies with rich and sustainable presentations of results will probably offer the best foundation for a proper synthesis. In my own experience, 10–20 primary studies with adequate information power may be feasible, while fewer primary studies will generally provide too little material for upcycling.

These are some of the reasons why practical modifications have been made to the analytical process prescribed by Noblit and Hare (Toye et al., 2014). In the project about the role of the NHD at the end of life, the synthesis was based on a sample of 14 primary studies (Fosse et al., 2014), while the synthesis of qualitative studies about stigma and obesity in health care used 13 primary studies (Malterud & Ulriksen, 2011). It is self-evident that procedures are different with a substantially larger sample than what Noblit and Hare describe. In both of these meta-ethnographies, the analysis sets out from identification of certain relevant themes. Other researchers have also chosen this route (Atkins et al., 2008; Riese et al., 2014).

If you decide on meta-ethnography as your preferred strategy, you will need more knowledge than what you will read in this book. You should approach the original references, supplemented with close reading of some articles where this method has been used (Noblit & Hare, 1988; Larun & Malterud, 2007; Malterud & Ulriksen, 2011; Dahl et al., 2013; Fosse et al., 2014). Campbell et al. (2011) argue that the method is constantly evolving and can hardly be taken as a standardized formula. Meta-methodical studies have however documented that meta-ethnography is often used as a reference in metasyntheses, without presenting sufficiently proper footprints as per Noblit and Hare's specifications (Bondas & Hall, 2007b; Dixon-Woods et al., 2007; Hannes & Macaitis, 2012; France et al., 2014; Thorne, 2017). In such cases, intersubjectivity and transparency will be jeopardized.

If you intend to modify the original method and refer to that choice in your method section, you must attend to the specific hallmarks of the method described above. If you want to deviate a great deal from the original specification, it is better to consider whether another method for synthesis is more suitable for you. However, we should all keep in mind that the method is merely your tool and not your aim. In becoming too preoccupied with procedures at the expense of interpretation, we might instrumentalize analysis, turn it into a technical exercise and forget the synthesis itself (Popay et al., 1998; Chamberlain, 2000; Thorne, 2015; Britten et al., 2017).

Other methods for qualitative metasynthesis

We find distinct traces of Noblit and Hare's meta-ethnography in most methods developed for qualitative metasynthesis. Some methods bear more pronounced imprints of the principles and procedures from the Cochrane SR tradition, and several methods resemble one another to a significant extent. Here, we take a brief look at three methods that have been used in studies beyond those of the methodology authors themselves.

Critical interpretive synthesis

Dixon-Woods et al. (2006) developed Critical interpretive synthesis as a method for qualitative metasynthesis. The authors take Noblit and Hare's meta-ethnography as their starting point, and the method bears several resemblances to that approach (Noblit & Hare, 1988). Furthermore, Critical interpretive synthesis follows several of the general rules for SRs that were not included in the original description of meta-ethnography presented above. In presenting Critical interpretive synthesis, the authors wanted to offer a methodical tool for upcycling and synthesizing research evidence independent of design, with the capacity to include both qualitative and quantitative primary studies in a single metasynthesis. The presentation of this method was illustrated by an example of research about accessibility for health care services among individuals from vulnerable population groups (Dixon-Woods et al., 2006).

Critical interpretive synthesis is intended for the synthesis of a sizable sample of primary studies. While Noblit and Hare's examples demonstrate the synthesis of just a few qualitative primary studies, Dixon-Woods et al. (2006) included 119 primary studies selected from an initial search that led to approximately 1,200 hits in their example. The authors recommend a purposive or theoretical sample comparable to those applied in qualitative studies in general, with relevance and maximal variation as essential criteria for inclusion. They demonstrate how their aim was inductively adjusted during the search and literature review stages. An appraisal of quality was also conducted, although with a high threshold for exclusion of studies with low quality. Data extraction was carried out in a pragmatic way with summaries of more extensive texts.

Like Noblit and Hare, the authors emphasize that Critical interpretive synthesis aims to develop new knowledge and novel concepts by means of interpretation, not just to describe and sum up existing research. As indicated by its name, Critical interpretive synthesis is a method intended for asking critical questions of assumptions widely taken for granted. Preparations for the study about accessibility of health care services for individuals from vulnerable population groups were therefore initiated by a critical assessment of whether consumption of health care services was an adequate measure of accessibility.

According to the critical perspective, Dixon-Woods et al. argue that Noblit and Hare's reciprocal translation analysis merely leads to summaries of knowledge from existing research, while refutational synthesis and lines-of-argument synthesis are necessary to achieve interpretation and synthesis beyond the descriptive level. In analysis, what distinguishes the individual primary studies from the subsequent logical arguments is therefore emphasized, inspired by the principles of *constant comparison* drawn from Grounded theory (Glaser & Strauss, 1967). *Candidacy* is an example of a substantive concept developed as an outcome of this synthesis. The analysis presented demonstrates how this concept offers insights into the preconditions for individuals' access to health care services, such as continuous negotiations, navigating the system, the permeability of the system when individuals present their candidacy for services and the adjudication carried out by professionals who either enable or inhibit the continued progress of candidacy (Dixon-Woods et al., 2006).

Laliberte Rudman et al. (2016) used Critical interpretive synthesis for a synthesis of research literature about risk and low-vision rehabilitation for older adults with age-related vision loss. They aimed to identify key guiding assumptions regarding risk and to discuss implications for what is and is not attended to in research and rehabilitation. The outcome of their literature search was 318 hits. After review, 83 were included for analysis. The authors found that risk based on assumptions aligned with a technico-scientific perspective is dominant, with risk conceptualized as an embodied, individual-level phenomenon that is to be determined and managed through objective screening and expert monitoring.

As a method for synthesis, Critical interpretive synthesis calls for thorough basic competence and skills in research and social science theories. Infrastructure support for the management and overview of sizeable amounts of literature and data is also necessary. When all these resources have been secured, the method can mediate important contributions to new understandings of illness and health. One challenge to implementation is that the explicit procedure for Critical interpretive synthesis has not been presented in great detail.

Thematic synthesis

Thematic synthesis was presented as a method for qualitative meta-synthesis by Thomas and Harden (2008). It is also based on meta-ethnography, buttressed by Grounded theory (Glaser & Strauss, 1967; Noblit & Hare, 1988). Thematic synthesis is also inspired by generic methods for thematic analysis of qualitative primary data (Braun & Clarke, 2006). The authors describe the following three steps of analysis: (1) systematic line-by-line *coding* of text from results sections, (2) organizing codes into a hierarchical structure exhibiting *descriptive themes* and (3) developing *analytic themes* by abstraction of the descriptive themes. In Thematic synthesis, the coding is supposed to accommodate translation and comparison across primary studies. The first two steps are compared to the reciprocal translation analysis found in meta-ethnography, while the last step is intended to lead to third-order concepts (Schutz, 1962; Britten et al., 2002; Barnett-Page & Thomas, 2009).

Sibeoni et al. (2017) used Thematic synthesis for a comparison and synthesis of the research literature about experiences of anorexia among adolescents, their families and health care professionals. The literature search produced 1,436 hits, and after review, 30 qualitative primary studies were included in the analysis. The authors found important disparities between the three stakeholders' understandings of causality and experiences, especially between the adolescents and the professionals, revealing challenges to developing a therapeutic alliance.

The description of this method has many similarities with the presentation of meta-ethnography above. One important difference, however, is that Thematic synthesis does not approach metaphors as a pivotal element of analysis. Another is the understanding of translation. While Noblit and Hare highlight the impact of meta-ethnography as a research method belonging to the interpretative paradigm, analysis and translation in Thematic synthesis may be not only inductive and data-driven but also deductive and theory-driven, with an epistemological basis in *objective realism* (Barnett-Page & Thomas, 2009).

Since analysis in Thematic synthesis emphasizes similarities between studies, the potential for demonstrating analytic contrasts and contradictions in the material is limited. This shortcoming is confirmed when Thomas and Harden argue that it is possible to close analysis with a presentation of the descriptive themes, if they can properly elucidate the aim of the study. The method is pragmatic with substantial feasibility but has been criticized for a lack of transparency in the analytic process and for its confined analytic ambitions (Dixon-Woods et al., 2005).

Realist synthesis

Realist synthesis (also referred to as Realist review) was introduced by Pawson et al. (2005) as a response to the critique of SRs from the Cochrane tradition, which were based on standardized effect studies with RCT designs that downplayed or even dismissed the social and cultural contexts. An important element of this critique is that SRs often sum up the effects of complex interventions without presenting sufficiently specific details about the interventions themselves and how they were implemented (Glasziou et al., 2008). Others point out that effect studies are often conducted in compound landscapes under varying conditions that cannot be completely controlled (Dobrow et al., 2004), with the consequence that it may be entirely misleading to ask only whether or not a particular intervention works (Petticrew, 2015).

With Realist synthesis, on the other hand, the question is not whether the intervention works but what works for whom under which conditions – how and why (Pawson et al., 2005). Realist reviews are driven by theory and seek to unpack the context-mechanism-outcome (CMO) relationship, thereby explaining examples of success, failure and various eventualities in between. The "realist" concepts refer to an epistemological position in which context and complexity are regarded as social realities that establish frames for people's conclusions and actions (Wong et al., 2013). The literature search strategy in Realist synthesis does not comply with the standard SR methodology. It rather resembles a purposive sample of the kind found in qualitative primary studies. The synthesis implies a systematic review of the relevant literature about theories to explain the mechanisms of the intervention in question, emphasizing the context (C) that may have released the relevant mechanisms (M) to achieve the desired outcomes (O). As opposed to other methods of metasynthesis, theories about the mode of operation – not the results from primary studies – are the major units of analysis in Realist synthesis.

Fernee et al. (2016) used Realist synthesis for a review of the research literature about wilderness therapy for groups of adolescents (12–18 years old) with mental health problems. The outcome of the literature search was 360 hits. After review, selected elements from seven qualitative studies about different programs for wilderness therapy were included. Analysis exploring CMO elements led to hypotheses about how the psychosocial context, the physical challenges and the everyday interaction in the group could combine to help challenge stereotypes so that the participants could get along with one another despite their problems with social relationships.

Realist synthesis is presented more like a logic and a strategy than a method of synthesis, with few details about the specific procedures to employ (Wong et al., 2013). This is a strategy in which social science competence and skills are necessary, and it may be difficult to fully understand since the concept and the method are applied in many different ways. If you want to use this strategy, it is therefore necessary to invest time and resources to approach the sources and pick up the theoretical foundation.

Reporting your study – writing the article

Most often, qualitative metasynthesis is reported as a research article published in a scientific journal. The text format is regulated by the house style of the specific journal to which the article is submitted. Composition and outline have many similarities with an article from a qualitative empirical primary study. The NOKC and other institutions affiliated with the Cochrane Collaboration present their SRs as extensive reports in a specific format. Below, we go through some special challenges that arise when writing a journal article about what we have done and what we have found using qualitative metasynthesis as a research method.

Elements in the article

The acronym *IMRAD* represents an outline with a set order: introduction, method, results and discussion (Sollaci & Pereira, 2004). Analogous outlines are used in academic writing in the social sciences (Major & Savin-Baden, 2010). A pertinent headline and a proper abstract can be absolutely decisive for whether others will read your article. Fosse's metasynthesis about the role of the NHD at the end of life (2014) was published in the journal Patient Education and Counseling with the title "End-of-life expectations and experiences among nursing home patients and their relatives – a synthesis of qualitative studies".

Independent of topic and method, an article in a journal for research in medicine or the health sciences starts out with an introductory *background section* that justifies the study's aim and sets the frames for the study. When presenting a qualitative metasynthesis, it is a challenge to write this section without anticipating the findings from your analysis (Saini & Shlonsky, 2012). On the one hand, you are supposed to demonstrate your familiarity with the topic. On the other, your introduction is expected to represent the knowledge base prior to your systematized approach. Take care not to "spend" in the introduction the articles that will later be your point of departure for analysis and synthesis and that the introduction does not reflect the literature search you conducted and will report as an essential element of your methodical strategy. I prefer to start the process of writing by working on the results section. Later, I can return to the introduction and try to compose this part of the text in a "pre-mode", demonstrating the state of the research literature about the topic before I completed my search and analysis. Having positioned the presentation of one's results makes it easier to decide on the composition of the introduction, method and discussion sections. For support, you can seek out some published metasyntheses to find a couple of articles where you think these matters have been successfully resolved.

In your *method section*, you describe the design, material, sample and analysis (see below).

The *results* section is the heart of your article. This is where you share and elaborate the endpoints from the analysis and synthesis. In Fosse's metasynthesis about the role of the NHD at the end of life (2014), the results section comprises about 40% of the article's text, making it a prominent pivot point. You will encounter some notable challenges in writing this section due to the fact that the primary studies are usually very dissimilar, with differences in terminology, publication format and information power in the results. This may be compared to the challenges encountered in a focus group study where the participants express themselves rather heterogeneously, with different degrees of accuracy and meaning content and where we may also have data from several group interviews with different moderators. In such cases, judgment must be used, emphasizing the assessment of the sustainability of the data and how far the findings can be extended in upcycling. We will emphasize the data that offers new knowledge and devote less space to what is already known. It is especially important not to refer each primary study in great detail – such presentations indicate that synthesis has not been very advanced. For a metasynthesis, synopsis and interpretation are our main assignments, as opposed to renarration and repetition. It will always be a challenge to present a synthesis containing sufficient amounts of new insight for others to be interested in reading it.

The *discussion section*, in which we reflect on the methodological strengths and weaknesses, compare our findings with previous research about the topic and discuss possible interpretations of our findings, will reflect our reflexivity and academic standards. Here, we are expected to highlight and discuss what is new as an outcome of our analysis. Finally, we pick up the threads and make connections, presented in conclusion and implications sections.

Oakley (2017) argues that systematic reviewing is a tool of democracy, and Lewin et al. (2018) suggest that qualitative evidence synthesis has the potential to widen the range of views and experiences represented in decision-making processes. Hence, disseminating the findings from a qualitative metasynthesis does not only mean addressing oneself to fellow researchers. Inspired by the Cochrane tradition of SRs, metasynthesis may also aim to speak to policymakers, civil servants and clinicians so that the evidence can be implemented in practice (Campbell et al., 2003; Atkins et al., 2008; Major & Savin-Baden, 2010). Still, new insight and understanding may be an adequate outcome of metasynthesis, without transformation to practical guidelines.

You will find that several challenges arise when you approach tangible implementation perspectives in a research article. Still, it is useful during the writing process to remind yourself that what you are writing is supposed to have meaning and lead to action beyond the academic world. For this purpose, Kvale's concepts of *communicative* and *pragmatic validity* may be useful (1996). The readability of your report will determine whether you have succeeded in developing knowledge that can be shared by others, and the utility of your knowledge will determine whether it will make a difference. The literary style of a research journal article is, however, far removed from what is suitable for such purposes, and often your published article will serve as a later point of departure for popularized, tailored and strategic dissemination.

Method, material and analysis

In qualitative studies, intersubjectivity and systematics are more relevant criteria than reproducibility (Malterud, 2001b; Wong, 2016). For qualitative synthesis, this has an impact on how we present the procedures we followed for searching and reviewing the literature and selecting the primary studies included (Tong et al., 2012). The reader expects to be able to imagine the path we followed and obtain insight into the important choices we have made. We will present search words, databases and time periods for the searches, account for our inclusion criteria and appraisal of primary studies and explain which considerations and additional strategies we have followed to strike the best possible balance between sensitivity and specificity in our search. However, it is not an aim that another researcher would reach exactly the same conclusions as ours.

Meta-methodical studies have criticized a general lack of transparency in qualitative metasyntheses, especially regarding analysis and synthesis (Bondas & Hall, 2007b; Dixon-Woods et al., 2007; France et al., 2014). It is thus important that you make explicit the criteria you followed for data extraction and selecting text segments for further analysis. If you made substantial compromises, you must first consider whether they were methodologically warranted and then describe, explain and discuss them (Tong et al., 2012). If you are a novice, you are better off choosing a method and following its procedures as closely as is feasible. At the beginning of the method presentation, you should let the reader see the method chosen for analysis and synthesis (Tong et al., 2012). In the text that follows, there should be no room for a reader to doubt that the method has been followed. In the discussion, you should reflect on alternative strategies and lay out the justifications for and consequences of your choices.

The process of analysis and synthesis can be illustrated by specific examples that make it easier for the reader to understand how you used the method to carry out the analysis and synthesis and develop the results you present. Give the reader examples of the kinds of empirical material you took as your point of departure and the moves you made to recognize connections, similarities and differences among the primary studies. It can also be useful to make clear how you understood vital concepts such as translation and metaphors and the impact of your understanding when you encountered the empirical data you extracted. As you begin to write about these issues, you will often discover that there are links in the analysis for which you cannot fully account. Take the time needed for reflection and finding the proper way of making this explicit in hindsight. Specific examples may contribute to insights in this regard.

In the article presenting the metasynthesis about stigma and obesity in the health care system we published the final version of the matrix (Malterud & Ulriksen, 2011). This approach may reveal the process more clearly than a table with codes, code groups and result categories, which can risk giving a misleading and linear impression of a process that was actually much more dynamic (Thorne, 2017). Often, however, the format of journal articles will limit the amount of what can be displayed. On the other hand, it is crucial to prioritize. Remember that examples only illustrate – but do not verify – the process. Do not forget that method is a means rather than a goal and ensure that your results are the core of your article (Thorne, 2017).

Synthesis and results

In all qualitative studies, including metasyntheses, the writing process constitutes the last stage of analysis. Preparing the text will either make it clear what have we found or, by contrast, demonstrate that we need to take a step backwards to tighten our grip on the results.

As you begin this step of elaborating your synthesis as text, you will realize the advantage of investing time and reflection in analysis and synthesis to understand what you have come up with and be able to share it with the reader. Another move that you will find useful at this stage is to organize your work so that you can maintain an overview of each primary study throughout the research process. This will enhance your opportunities to return to the empirical material if you need to check, augment or adjust the text when presenting your results and accommodate the context in its entirety (Thorne, 2017). This is also a good reason to limit the number of primary studies in your sample.

In an article reporting a qualitative metasynthesis, the presentation of results will ideally display the endpoints of analysis and synthesis in a format that deepens the reader's understanding of what we have found in an interesting and convincing way. At this point, it is far from sufficient to simply reproduce the primary studies we have read. Major and Savin-Baden (2010) recommend that you organize the presentation of your results as a kind of story that, in a substantive way, states the reasons for, expands on and disseminates the outcome of the synthesis. In presenting the evidence of your synthesis, the researcher takes responsibility to speak on behalf of both the authors and the participants in the primary studies, and the metasynthesis therefore necessarily reflects several different realities and experiences (Major & Savin-Baden, 2010). This is not fundamentally different from the situation we encounter when we write the results section in a qualitative interview study, where we are also supposed to take care of key epistemological conditions from social constructionism in interpretation and reporting (Lock & Strong, 2010).

Major and Savin-Baden (2010) list six alternative principles that can be used for designing the results section: (1) the (often chronological) logic of the story; (2) the natural sequence of the process, which is not necessarily linear; (3) the concepts in a hierarchical structure (superior first, then inferior); (4) starting with the most important results; (5) starting with the simplest results; (6) using a theory-driven approach. Independent of priority and order, the presentation of results should always appear as *thick descriptions* (Geertz, 2000) that are clearly anchored in the empirical basis of the analysis (Major & Savin-Baden, 2010).

There are several alternative ways of fulfilling this requirement in practice. Do not make it too complicated.

Table 3.3 illustrates how such result categories can be developed, all with reference to articles from four metasyntheses in which I have been involved (Larun & Malterud, 2007; Malterud & Ulriksen, 2011; Dahl et al., 2013; Fosse et al., 2014). These four metasyntheses are based on literature searches with between 667 and 834 unique hits, which after review for relevance and quality led to the inclusion of 13 to 20 primary studies for analysis and synthesis.

For the results from a qualitative metasynthesis to stand out as something more than the outcome of a descriptive, thematic analysis, your result categories should arise from a convincing and revealing synthesis. With these categories, you can proliferate your translation of metaphors from the different themes, expressing something more

Table 3.3 Examples of result categories.

First author (year): topic	Results categories
Larun (2007): *Chronic fatigue syndrome*	• Symptom experiences and consequences for everyday life • Identity • Strategies for coping
Malterud (2011): *Obesity, stigma and responsibility in health care*	• Apparently appropriate advice, perhaps well intended, yet perceived as patronizing • Abnormal bodies cannot be incorporated in the medical systems – exclusion consequently happens • Customary standards for interpersonal respect are legitimately surpassed – contempt as if deserved
Dahl (2013) *Lesbian families' experiences with health care providers in the birthing context*	• Encountering and managing overt and covert prejudice • Confidence can be created when professionals present knowledge and support • Disclosure of sexual orientation – important, but risky unless you are in charge of context • Accepting the lesbian family by recognizing both mothers
Fosse (2014): *End-of-life expectations and experiences among nursing home patients*	• When health personnel anticipate and recognize patients' needs for symptom relief, dignity may be preserved and family members feel relieved • Proxy decision-making in the face of uncertainty is painful for the family • Relatives or doctors do not always recognize patient preferences at the end of life

and something other than the sum of their parts (Tong et al., 2012). You can elaborate additional nuances of the overall synthesis in the discussion of results when you emphasize what is new in your study compared to existing research and discuss your contribution with the support of selected theoretical perspectives.

A relevant substantive theory supporting your analysis may make it easier for you to refine your results and contribute something that is not already known (Malterud, 2016). In the metasynthesis about lesbian families encountering the maternity ward, Dahl included Plummer's theory of intimate citizenship to better understand how cultural attitudes towards non-heterosexual relationships can influence how people are encountered in a sensitive situation (Plummer, 2003; Dahl et al., 2013). In this way, attention could be drawn to the social context of the birthing experiences rather than individual reactions and experiences. To be a family in labour disturbing the heteronormative pattern of habits and expectations leads to experiences that differ from those who belong to the majority in this context. This study gives an example of the impact of theoretical perspectives for a synthesis to deliver more than the results of each primary study included.

Try to craft a writing style in which you refer in the results section to those primary studies that provided substantial contributions to the different themes and their various elements. If the primary studies in your sample contain pertinent quotations, you may use them to illustrate your result categories (Tong et al., 2012). Just remember that – as in any qualitative study – quotations are neither proof nor documentation of the credibility of the results. The role of the quotations is to offer material support to what your analytic text describes.

It has been argued that the textual presentation of results should be accompanied by tables or figures (Major & Savin-Baden, 2010; France et al., 2014). Such a standard resembles the rules of the 1980s, which held that qualitative studies conducted using Grounded theory should be published only if their main findings had been summed up as a diagram (Wilson & Hutchinson, 1996). Models with boxes and arrows or hierarchical tree structures can certainly help by visualizing the most important connections, but they can also convey an impression that the author is not capable of expressing the main points in words.

I have found the general strategies for writing up qualitative primary studies to be useful when I report a qualitative metasynthesis. I organize the results section with the "story" told by the analysis of each main theme presented as different subsections of the results section, often with a few lines in which I present the major aspects of each main theme as the outcome of the synthesis. This writing strategy requires you to have accomplished the synthesis for the result categories for each theme rather than only an overarching synopsis. However, it is also important to consider how the different results can be translated together into a comprehensive understanding of what has been found. The analytic text in the results section will visualize and establish as plausible the content of meaning in each result category, which may be built up with subgroups (see Table 3.2). Here, we have developed the third-order concept "Apparently appropriate advice, perhaps well intended, yet perceived as patronizing" into a synthesis presented as analytical text illustrated by a few selected quotations (see Frame 3.1).

Apparently appropriate advice, perhaps well intended – yet perceived as patronizing.

Results from the included primary studies presented a broad range of accounts about seemingly adequate attitudes and recommendations from doctors and nurses regarding obesity and health (Brown & Thompson, 2007; Brown et al., 2006; Diaz, Mainous, & Pope, 2007; Epstein & Ogden, 2005; Merrill & Grassley, 208; Reed, 2003; Rogge et al., 2004; Thomas, Hyde, Karunaratne, Kausman, & Komesaroff, 2008; Wright, 1998). Female nurses expressed a strongly held belief that fat is unhealthy, particularly in relation to coronary heart disease, so that they felt they ought to persuade women to lose unhealthy fat (Wright, 1998). For this purpose, they would suggest exercise and dietary adjustments, yet they expressed various levels of discomfort related to counselling on such a sensitive topic (Brown & Thompson, 2007; Wright, 1998). Primary care nurses tried to steer a balanced course between factors of personal responsibility and factors beyond the control of the individual, while declaring that they took care to avoid stereotypes or overtly simplistic explanations (Brown & Thomposon, 2007). Strategies presented by doctors included maintaining a good relationship with the patients, trying to locate the weight problem in the broader context of their lives, despite not having a solution, and offering an understanding of the problems associated with obesity (Epstein & Ogden, 2005). Yet, there were several examples of descriptions where patients' efforts were presented in degrading terms. A British general practitioner (GP) said about one of his patients:

> She is a woman who has had a sort of fairly appalling diet, clues really about…what a calorie is… (Epstein & Ogden, 2005).

Patients, on the other hand, described their ongoing persistence of trying to control or lose weight, in general from their early teens (Thomas et al., 2008). From numerous experiences of unsuccessful dieting, they felt defeated by their weight and their failed attempts to control it, yet they refused to give up (Merrill & Grassley, 2008). They blamed themselves for being unable to stick to or continue with a weight loss plan, rather the diet (Thomas et al., 2008).

Participants in the studies included in our analysis presented different examples of communication perceived as insensitive, which had hardly been helpful (Brown et al., 2006). Providers who repeatedly pointed out that the patient's weight was a problem, without providing practical advice and support, might raise awareness but little more (Brown et al., 2006; Wright, 1998). Patients also complained that providers attributed any problem their weight, without checking the associations (Brown et al., 2006; Merrill & Grassley, 2008).

Addressing the problem as if there was a simple solution that had nor occurred to the patient was experienced as humiliating (Merrill & Grassley, 2008; Reed, 2003; Rogge et al., 2004; Wright 1998). A large US woman, considering bariatric surgery, refers the recommendations her GP gave her, where she should just drink more water and push myself away from the table I would think to myself, wow; if only I had thought of that before! (Reed, 2003).

Frame 3.1 Example of how a result category can be presented.
Source: Malterud and Ulriksen, 2011.

Transparency in reporting qualitative metasyntheses

Guidelines and checklists provide norms for reporting SRs and quantitative meta-analyses (Liberati et al., 2009), but the principles and procedures from this tradition cannot simply be transferred into qualitative metasynthesis. Tong et al. (2012) developed a framework suited to qualitative methods and intended to enable better reporting of this type of SR. A group of researchers with extensive practical experiences using these methods conducted a systematic literature search, identifying 381 relevant articles published between 1994 and 2011. Taking the methodology literature as their point of departure, they developed a pilot version of a checklist that was tested for a purposive sample of the articles and then revised.

The final version of the checklist, "Enhancing Transparency in Reporting the Synthesis of Qualitative Research" *(ENTREQ)*, consists of 21 questions in 5 domains: (1) introduction, (2) methods and methodology, (3) literature search and selection, (4) appraisal and (5) synthesis of findings (Tong et al., 2012). The authors state that they spent between 5 and 20 minutes reviewing and assessing each article with the ENTREQ checklist. It has, however, been argued that ENTREQ is too generic (France et al., 2014). The authors themselves express certain reservations regarding the validation of the checklist (Tong et al., 2012). Nevertheless, the checklist can be useful to draw attention to aspects of the writing process deserving special attention, independent of which analysis method you have used to conduct the qualitative metasynthesis.

The American Psychological Association recently presented detailed reporting standards for qualitative research, including Qualitative Meta-Analysis Article Reporting Standards *(QMARS)* (Levitt et al., 2018). The authors point out that they do not suggest that every element they have advanced is relevant in every study, adding that they expect that qualitative reporting standards will continue to shift and change.

4 Theoretical and methodological challenges

Qualitative methods encounter evidence-based medicine

Transparency and systematic approaches are essential criteria for scholarly conduct using qualitative research methods. Comparable standards are applicable to evidence-based medicine (EBM) as developed and elaborated within the Cochrane tradition. We might thus imagine that qualitative metasynthesis, staged as a systematic review (SR) of qualitative studies, would be a natural meeting point for these two methodological traditions. That is correct, but there are also several important distinctions that result from the different paradigms that support the two traditions. We will therefore face several significant challenges requiring reflexivity and methodological skills, and we will also be obliged to make some pragmatic compromises.

Scientific paradigms

Ontology is a concept from the philosophy of science that refers to how we understand the world and reality. *Epistemology* is the analogous concept for advancing knowledge about the world and reality. Consistency between ontology and epistemology is hence a logical prerequisite for scientific knowledge (Malterud, 2019). How we recognize the world will determine relevant and valid approaches for studying the world and understanding reality, and the other way round: the perspectives embedded in our knowledge about the world will have an impact on how we understand and perceive it.

Normative assumptions establish the historical, social and cultural frames for the development of knowledge and regulate what we label as scientific (Kvale, 1996; Alvesson & Sköldberg, 2009). We ordinarily take much of this for granted without questioning why it is so, how it is shaped in practice or whether it will necessarily remain as it is.

The philosopher of science Thomas Kuhn (1962) called such funda-mental assumptions about the world and our knowledge of the world scientific *paradigms*.

The *positivist paradigm* enjoys high standing in the biomedical re-search tradition, based on ontological assumptions about a stable, predictable and governable reality (Crotty, 2003). The epistemological impact of a positivist understanding is that observations and measure-ments processed with deductive strategies are relevant research meth-ods that lead to objective facts. Quantitative research methods such as statistics and epidemiology belong to the positivist paradigm, and the methodology for SRs has been developed within this tradition.

The *interpretative paradigm* is based on humanist traditions in which reality is understood to be embedded in subjective experiences, mean-ings and interpretations in social and historical contexts (Malterud, 2001b). The epistemological consequences are that such phenomena can be studied by means of talk, interaction and text and further pro-cessed with inductive strategies that reveal different versions of reality that depend on position and perspective (Crotty, 2003). Qualitative research methods like phenomenology or ethnography belong to this paradigm. The 14 qualitative primary studies in Fosse's metasynthesis (2014) about the role of the nursing home doctor (NHD) at the end of life deal with subjective experiences from patients and relatives, in-cluding decision processes, preferences, symptom experiences, dignity and advance care directives – issues for which counting and measure-ments have little or no relevance.

Common features, differences and opposites

There are several indispensable common features in quantitative and qualitative research methods. Reflexivity, relevance and validity are major criteria in all research (Malterud, 2001b), and I find it incor-rect and detrimental to claim that one is inherently better than the other. In medicine and health sciences, there is a need for a diversity of knowledge. It is necessary to develop dialogues in which different concepts of knowledge complement one another rather than being re-garded as irretrievably incompatible opposites. At the same time, it is important to choose a research method with appropriate epistemolog-ical agreement with what we want to study.

Taken together, the positivist and interpretative paradigms imply cer-tain ontological and epistemological contradictions that we must face when qualitative and quantitative research traditions interact. Quali-tative metasynthesis is one such arena (Wong, 2016; Malterud, 2019).

Pettycrew (2015) asks some basic questions about the methodology of SRs when employed in qualitative metasynthesis. The contradictions have an impact on how research methods are operationalized and what is considered valid knowledge, especially when it comes to strategies for analysis, understanding of transferability and objectivity and about the impact of reflexivity (Malterud, 1993, 2016; Popay et al., 1998).

As a researcher, you are supposed to have appropriate basic knowledge of and skills in the different methods so that you can choose the method best suited to exploring the problem you have chosen. If you want to know more about the prevalence and distribution of diabetes, you should choose an epidemiological method. If you want to know more about the effects of drug therapy for diabetes, you should choose a randomized controlled trial (RCT) or an SR of RCTs. If you want to know more about the experiences and goals of individuals with diabetes, you should choose a qualitative method. If you want to recapitulate the evidence reported in previous qualitative studies, you should choose metasynthesis.

Scholarly competence requires that you not only master methodological skills but also be familiar with and respect the epistemological assumptions underlying different research methods. Qualitative metasynthesis, as this research tradition has been developed and as I present it in this book, is a qualitative research method. Nevertheless, several of its technical procedures, especially concerning searching and reviewing literature, originate from the positivist roots of the Cochrane tradition and are conceptualized as facts, representativity and objectivity (Popay et al., 1998). How can these pursuits best be combined without creating overly problematic compromises?

Social anthropology and metasynthesis

These are the kinds of challenges that Riese et al. (2014) take as their point of departure in discussing whether qualitative metasynthesis is consistent with the tradition and methodology of social anthropology. These authors suggest that the primary studies included in a metasynthesis can be compared to an anthropologist's cases, and the authors of the primary studies may be considered key informants. For metasynthesis to be appropriate as a research method for anthropology, Riese et al. join many others in supposing as a precondition that analysis will lead to the development of new understanding and theory and not mere aggregation and renarration.

The authors argue that constant comparison, a core strategy in qualitative metasynthesis, corresponds well with the research traditions of social anthropology. The point of departure must be a critical appraisal of whether the material from the primary studies provides sufficiently sustainable presentations of not only results but also the context necessary to upcycle the findings as an appropriate synthesis (Popay et al., 1998; Geertz, 2000; Saini & Shlonsky, 2012; Riese et al., 2014; Malterud, 2019). There are also warnings against including too many primary studies in the analysis, which may cause the researcher to lose sight of the big picture. These are vital reservations, and you need not be a social anthropologist to approve of them. In the process of Fosse's metasynthesis about the role of the NHD at the end of life, we confirmed by our own experience that it was possible to preserve an overview of the 14 primary studies included, but we also learned how important it was to be thoroughly familiar with each study and assess the impact of the context in which each was conducted (Fosse et al., 2014). This was even more challenging in the metasynthesis about Chronic fatigue syndrome/Myalgic encephalopathy (CFS/ME) experiences, which included 20 primary studies (Larun & Malterud, 2007). Furthermore – and unfortunately – qualitative studies do not always report sufficient information about their contexts.

These considerations demonstrate how we can link up with some of the challenges in the point of intersection between the paradigms. It is certainly feasible to take note of certain academic conditions or critical questions without then having to dismiss any methodological moves drawn from SRs and the meta-analysis of quantitative studies. We can use our scholarly competence to assess the preconditions for and consequences of different choices in the research process and manage them in a pragmatic fashion. As long as we share and provide good grounds for our concerns, we can attend to intersubjectivity and allow the reader room for access and critique (Malterud, 1993). Still, we will not stint on basic methodological principles.

A complete and independent literature review?

The standard methodology for search and appraisal of primary studies for an SR implies the assumption that it is possible and appropriate to reach a definite and complete answer to the question of what evidence about a certain topic exists at a given point in time. Moreover, the recommended procedures for appraising relevance and quality in the literature search represent norms implying that independent assessments will strengthen the credibility of what we do and what we find. For metasynthesis, which is rooted in qualitative research methods, these assumptions represent dilemmas associated with how we think about objectivity and evidence.

Situated knowledges

Donna Haraway is a feminist and philosopher of science with a background in mammalian biology. She questions the traditional understanding of *objectivity*, understood as the ontological and epistemological assumptions that it is possible to see everything from nowhere, that knowledge can be independent of premises or standpoint. She calls this perspective "the *God trick* of seeing everything from nowhere" (Haraway, 1991). Haraway's arguments sustain my wariness about research methods – whether qualitative or quantitative – that claim to show us "reality as it actually is."

Haraway compares the view of the researcher with animals' faculty of vision, which is their instrument to catch sight of what is of interest. We are speaking about actively sensing systems with determined and limited scope, being an integrated part of the animals themselves. The one who sees and the one being seen are both active subjects. Haraway argues that research and academic knowledge can be judged using a similar logic. The way the view of the researcher is positioned will determine what is seen – there is no position from which anybody can see the totality in an unambiguous and universal way with objective distance, as implied by the God trick (Haraway, 1991).

Furthermore, Haraway argues that translations are always interpretative, critical and incomplete. Still, she is no radical postmodern social constructionist declaring that all versions of reality are equal. As a feminist, she is aware that critique of structural and normative issues is needed, with some perspectives reflecting reality in a more relevant way than others. For example, it is an important difference to observe something from below as opposed to above. Still, the perspective from below is not always the best or the most relevant one.

As a point of departure for an alternative understanding of objectivity, Haraway presents the concept of *situated knowledges* (1991), using the plural to emphasize that we are speaking about several possible alternatives of knowledge as opposed to a single, universal truth. In saying so, she promotes a view of objectivity in which the knower is acknowledged and assigned responsibility. As a researcher, I must take responsibility for what I see by explicating and reflecting upon my premises and conditions – my *positioning*, which determines the situating of the knowledge I develop.

It is therefore pointless to try to eliminate your own position – in fact, quite the opposite is true. You should announce and argue for your position, because it is an integrated element of what you see (Kelly et al., 2015). This perspective fits well with how reflexivity is understood and valued in qualitative research (Finlay, 2008; Alvesson &

Sköldberg, 2009). Supported by Haraway's arguments, we could say that the question is not whether the researcher influences the process, but how much and in what ways (Malterud, 1993; Saini & Shlonsky, 2012; Ioannidis, 2016).

We expect researchers to acknowledge their preconceptions and footprints and examine their impact in the pursuit of knowledge, realizing that the window being opened by analysis will only give access to a limited and incomplete part of reality (Kelly et al., 2015). In Fosse's metasynthesis (2014) about the role of the NHD at the end of life, all members of the research team were experienced clinicians who shared a conception that death is an important part of life that should not be rendered invisible. This standpoint certainly had an influence on the process of analysis and is therefore included in the methodology discussion. In the metasynthesis about lesbian families encountering the maternity ward, the research team included four people with different professional backgrounds (medical doctor, health visitor, midwife) and sexual orientations (Dahl et al., 2013). This probably contributed to other perspectives on relevant data and thus a different situating of knowledge than if the research team had consisted solely of, for example, lesbian midwives.

These perspectives from the philosophy of science serve as a starting point for critique of the idea that the literature search in an SR will have the capacity to establish a complete and independent overview of research knowledge about a certain topic. That understanding of knowledge is not compliant with the basic criteria of qualitative research methods (MacLure, 2005; Malterud, 2019), but what, in that case, are the alternatives?

Cherry picking

As readers, we expect an SR to reveal a selection of research results that demonstrates the scope of research literature, presents different perspectives on the aim of our study, satisfies scholarly standards and serves as the outcome of a process that can withstand close scrutiny. If those expectations are to be met, we cannot simply decide on a sample of publications chosen to support our own points of view. *Cherry picking* implies that we select and include what suits us best and put the rest aside. Cherry picking does not indicate critical reflection.

By conducting a systematic literature search and a critical review, we will establish a sample of empirical data that is suitable for analysis and synthesis. Neither coincidence nor luck will guarantee a sample to be sustainable for upcycling. Therefore, the literature search in an

SR is expected to be documented by search terms, search sources and inclusion criteria (see Chapter 2). These procedures can counteract cherry picking and ensure transparency and critique. This is especially important for topics about which there is disagreement as to the kind of evidence on which to rely, as is true, for example, of research about CFS/ME (Larun & Malterud, 2007).

For a qualitative primary study, we use other principles for sampling than in a quantitative study, where completeness, independence, representativity and standardization stand out as indispensable criteria. In a qualitative study, on the other hand, we recognize and emphasize the researcher's involvement in the process when we establish a purposive sample. Supported by theory, experience and previous research, we compose a sample of qualitative data which is specific, relevant and diverse as to the phenomena we intend to explore (Kuzel, 1999; Patton, 2015). These are systematic and transparent sampling processes, something very different from cherry picking. Principles of theoretical sampling drawn from Grounded theory may also be applied (Finfgeld-Connett, 2018). Similar principles can be assigned to qualitative metasynthesis.

The standard criteria for establishing the sample for an SR have been developed in research traditions where quantitative studies are summed up by means of statistical methods. In that context, the aim of a complete, representative and homogeneous sample can be desirable and at least partly feasible. For a sample intended for qualitative metasynthesis, however, such assumptions are problematic (Booth, 2016; Malterud, 2019). In qualitative studies, rich and diverse data offering thick descriptions are more important than representativity and standardization.

Several researchers discuss the possibilities of using purposive samples in qualitative metasynthesis, replacing a search strategy intended to include the whole (Dixon-Woods et al., 2006; Saini & Shlonsky, 2012; Booth, 2016; Britten et al., 2017). However, a comprehensive search will always somehow remain a precondition, because a purposive sample requires a qualified overview of the literature (Atkins et al., 2008; Sandelowski, 2012). The more creative the search strategy we choose, the more complicated it will be to report it. So far, the methodology literature about qualitative metasyntheses offers no specific answers as to how best to resolve this challenge in practice.

Saturation has been suggested as a criterion to appraise the size and composition of a sample (Petticrew, 2015; Booth, 2016). There are, however, many challenges related to this concept, not least because it is rooted in a particular methodological tradition (Grounded theory). *Information power* may therefore be better suited to this purpose, because this concept calls on us to take a stand on selected properties of the actual study to assess whether we need a large or a small sample (Malterud et al., 2016b). Elements contributing to high information power can, separately or taken together, imply that the number of participants in a primary study can be limited. In a similar fashion, primary studies contributing to high informational power may, separately or taken together, imply that the number of primary studies in the sample for a metasynthesis can be limited. Such an appraisal may also include sustainability, a term used here in the sense of evidence that has appropriate capacity for upcycling.

Finding the needle in the haystack

Norwegian Knowledge Centre for the Health Services (NOKC) advises that a well-conducted literature search is important to identify all relevant research worldwide about a certain topic (Nasjonalt kunnskapssenter for helsetjenesten, 2015), because only then will it be possible to give a reliable answer about the effect of an intervention. The technology offers endless possibilities of undertaking comprehensive digital literature searches. When this is combined with an ambition that the search will serve as the foundation for a complete overview of the literature, we may end up with vast number of hits in need of screening with established procedures before the synthesis itself can be initiated. In the worst cases, technical exercises are given priority over interpretation and synthesis (Thorne, 2015; Britten et al., 2017; Thorne, 2017).

Simply put, the largest sample is not the best point of departure. MacLure (2005) points out that only a small proportion of the hits from the literature search survives screening to be included among the primary studies – 0.3% is reported as a typical example of the rate of survival. She asks whether these procedures to find the needle in the haystack are actually well suited to the purpose at hand. At this point we may also be reminded of Haraway's argument (1991) that knowledge is always partial.

There appears to be a tendency for metasyntheses to be conducted with steadily larger samples of primary studies (see Chapter 3 (France et al., 2014)). At the same time, the point of departure for selection – the size of the literature search – is also increasing. For example, O'Rourke et al. conducted a metasynthesis about quality of life among individuals with dementia based on 11 primary studies identified after a review of 5,625 hits from the search (H. M. O'Rourke et al., 2015). This means that only 0.2% were included, while 99.8% (N = 5,614) were first screened and then discarded. Fosse's metasynthesis about the role of the NHD at the end of life (2014) included 14 primary studies identified after reviewing 505 hits. In this case, 2.8% were included, with 97.2% (N = 491) discarded. Given such a low inclusion percentage or survival rate, we may ask whether the screening process justifies the resources needed and whether it is possible to make sufficiently steady eye contact to retain an appropriate and relevant level of accuracy in the review process (White, 2001). Brunton et al. (2017) criticize as myth the notion that it is possible to identify every single relevant study for any SR, and Campbell et al. (2011) comment that the results of a synthesis will hardly change radically if some studies are overlooked.

A persistent problem in qualitative studies is the analysis of extensive samples that have only limited relevance (Kvale, 1996). In such studies, the research question is often broad and fuzzy, and the results are not very distinct or original. There is an analogous logic for qualitative metasynthesis. With a fine-toothed comb we will struggle with too much contamination, while a less exhaustive search will provide an insufficient number of relevant results (Egger et al., 2003; Booth, 2016). The information power of the empirical material for our metasynthesis may be strengthened with a focused research question and distinct and appropriate search terms.

Independent appraisals or bias?

The methodology literature for SRs emphasizes that screening and appraisal of the results from the literature search should be conducted independently by at least two researchers (Egger et al., 2003; Liberati et al., 2009; Saini & Shlonsky, 2012; Nasjonalt kunnskapssenter for helsetjenesten, 2015). Similar recommendations are given for data extraction from the primary studies included. These principles reflect the idea that two researchers who follow the same procedure ought to reach the same conclusion, and that any such outcome will not be influenced by the people who carried out the search procedure. *Independence* is assumed to counteract *bias*, which leads to undesirable or unintended skewness in the research. Under this epistemological logic, *reproducibility* is selected as a criterion for objectivity in a traditional sense (Booth, 2016; Wong, 2016), which is actually what Haraway (1991) calls the God trick.

Within the interpretative paradigm, reflexive subjectivity is a basic precondition to avoid prejudiced interpretations (Popay et al., 1998). Our procedures and analyses require that we attend responsibly and reflexively to the question of how the researcher influences the process and the consequences of that influence (Finlay, 2008). When two researchers have opposing views on a matter, such as whether a primary study is to be included for synthesis, it conveys the situation that several different alternatives may be valid at the same time, not necessarily that one is wrong or that the criteria are faulty. Such oppositions, in fact, serve as a good point of departure for dialogue and negotiation that may lead to important contributions that sharpen the research question and criteria for inclusion. They are not necessarily indications of deficient appraisal accuracy.

When the researcher is not sufficiently open-minded towards oppositions or contradictions, or when coincidence or a lack of systematicity is allowed to rule, skewness that is undesirable in a qualitative study may appear. Hence, intersubjectivity and reflexivity are vital tools to practice Haraway's situated knowledges, in the sense of interpretative research that acknowledges and takes a stand on the role and motives of the researcher. The purpose is not to eliminate the impact of the researcher's influence. On the contrary, it should be rendered visible and its consequences made subject to discussion. The epistemological logic of qualitative metasyntheses therefore takes account of dialogue and transparency rather than independence and neutrality (Malterud, 2019).

At this point, the methodological literature still lacks specific guidance on how best to undertake and report this in practice. Therefore, my recommendation is that we exercise critical judgment regarding the recommended practices, considering which ones actually fit best into an interpretative and qualitative logic. To downscale search procedures and choose alternative moves, high levels of transparency and reflexivity are required to offer appropriate access for understanding the process (Sandelowski, 2012; Petticrew, 2015).

Which evidence is the best evidence?

Several concerns will determine the validity and trustworthiness of evidence from processes in which we identify, organize and assemble the results from research conducted by somebody else. Regardless of whether the method is statistical meta-analysis or qualitative metasynthesis, the numerous links in the chain of translation may lead to results that are unclear or even misleading. What is needed to develop sustainable evidence, and to what degree can we trust the results of the synthesis? For a qualitative metasynthesis, the quality of data, the way they are processed and the purpose of the knowledge development will establish the limits for the kinds of results we can present and what uses they can serve.

The evidence hierarchy

EBM includes methods for summing up research knowledge (incoming evidence) in the format of SRs (outgoing evidence) as the foundation for decisions in health care policy and practice. In this book, I use the term *evidence* as a unified concept covering research results, independent of topic, method or quality. A crucial element drawn from the EBM tradition is to appraise the scientific quality of any such evidence.

Initially, the study target for such reviews was effect studies. It was for this purpose that standards assessing which kind of research design provides the best evidence were established. The *evidence hierarchy* was first presented by a Canadian committee in a review of the effect of interventions proposed for routine annual check-ups (Canadian Task Force on the Periodic Health Examination, 1979). Evidence was ranked after research design as follows:

1   Evidence obtained from at least one properly randomized controlled trial.
2   a   Evidence obtained from well-designed cohort or case-control analytic studies, preferably from more than one centre or research group.
     b   Evidence obtained from comparisons between times or places with or without the interventions, including dramatic results in uncontrolled experiments.
3   Opinions from respected authorities, based on clinical experience, descriptive studies or reports of expert committees.

In this context, results from cohort studies and case-control studies were deemed to be evidence of inherently lower quality than RCT results. These norms gained broad approval and (appropriately) set the methodological gold standard to answer the question of whether or not an intervention works. Gradually, attention within the EBM movement shifted from critical appraisal of individual studies to summing up effect studies and meta-analyses, where evidence from RCTs again ranked first (Cochrane, 1989).

The evidence hierarchy has often been presented in the format of a pyramid, with the highest-quality evidence on top and the lowest-quality evidence at the bottom (Shaneyfelt, 2016). In 2006, a research group at Dartmouth College and Yale University presented an evidence pyramid based on the hierarchy from the 1979 Canadian committee (Glover et al., 2006) (see Figure 4.1). This pyramid gained

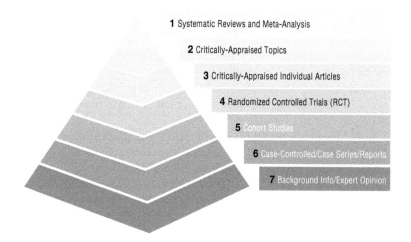

Figure 4.1 The EBM pyramid adapted from Dartmouth College and Yale
     University (Glover et al., 2006).
Source: Redrawn from EMB-pyramiden, Bygger på EBM Pyramid fra Dartmouth
College og Yale University, 2017.

widespread attention and was developed as a tool for EBM training
and practice. It features a ranking of evidence after research design,
with RCTs better than cohort studies, which are better than case-
control studies and various types of case studies. The pyramid does
not explicitly assess the value of qualitative studies, but in this context
qualitative studies are most similar to the case studies located near the
bottom of the pyramid.

A universal gold standard?

Miscellaneous research designs provide evidence of different cur-
rency and credibility for various purposes. When answering questions
about whether an intervention works, we prefer evidence from an RCT
rather than from a focus group study. Ideally, we would want a systematic review of all relevant RCTs. Similarly, when answering questions
about experiences or adventures, evidence from a focus group study is
preferred to an RCT.

It is not problematic that these kinds of questions are simplified
when they are communicated in an educational format. It is, however, a serious problem that the Canadian evidence hierarchy and the
pyramid from Dartmouth and Yale have contributed to the idea of a

universal gold standard that ranks different kinds of evidence and research design, independent of nature of the research question.

Most probably, I believe, the authors of the original evidence hierarchies have taken for granted a reference to effect studies. Over the
years, the need to refer explicitly to that kind of study has slowly but
surely disappeared. Different evidence pyramids have gained widespread attention and contributed to supporting the prevailing understanding of a universal evidence hierarchy for medical and health
research. It is, for example, still argued that an RCT design offers
better evidence than qualitative research methods without specification of the preconditions for and purposes of the deliveries of knowledge obtained through the various methods (Loder et al., 2016). This
is in stark contrast to Sackett and Wennberg's insistence (1997) that
the choice of method must be a consequence of a study's aim, meaning that no method can ever be inherently superior. Oakley (2017)
asserts that what matters is the question, and then the answer, emphasizing that the method must comply with the question.

In many academic environments, qualitative studies are still ranked
on the universal bottom position when we ask whether we can trust
evidence from this kind of study. For researchers who use qualitative
methods, such standpoints are all too familiar. Unfortunately, we still
may find that editors and reviewers will dismiss a qualitative study
by referring to the lack of a representative sample, a control group,
confidence intervals or standardized procedures, as if the preferred
research design is always an RCT.

Qualitative metasynthesis includes critical appraisal of incoming and
outgoing evidence, in which we are supposed to take a stand on whether
the results are sustainable – on how they can be compiled, interpreted
and upcycled (Gough et al., 2017a; Malterud, 2019). There are certainly
qualitative studies of high and low scientific standards, but for qualitative
research methods, we simply cannot talk in the same way about a clear
hierarchy of evidence. First, it makes no sense to use criteria developed
for summing up effect studies and, second, the study aim and context will
determine which of several possible qualitative designs is most appropriate. When we study experiences and attitudes, for example, qualitative
interview studies are more suitable than qualitative observational studies.

It is therefore necessary to involve preconditions and context when
assessing which design can offer the best possible evidence, given the
study's actual purpose (Malterud, 2019). The research method must be
determined in light of the research question, after which the quality
and scope of the results can be considered. For example, it is difficult to
imagine that an RCT or a meta-analysis of RCTs would be relevant to

or a realistic way of conducting an exploration of expectations and experiences associated with the role of the NHD at the end of life (2014). Methodological diversity may well result in sustainable evidence and a broad view of knowledge for practice. Qualitative metasynthesis is an important tool that should not escape critical assessment.

Appraisal of specific evidence must, however, be conducted from premises other than solely those referred to in the original evidence pyramid, which is still alive. Also in the Cochrane environment, there is an increasing recognition that the methodology for SRs of effect studies does not embody a universal gold standard that applies to all kinds of research questions. This recognition has been rendered concrete, for example, in the development of methods for SRs of diagnostic tests (Whiting et al., 2011) and is reinforced by the increasing interest in mixed methods and qualitative metasyntheses (Noyes & Lewin, 2011; Lewin et al., 2012).

Grading of evidence

With SRs intended to be the basis for developing recommendations and guidelines, we need to know whether an intervention is effective and whether we should consider the estimate of effect size to be rigorous or whether new studies are likely to change it. But even when the methodological rules of the game are followed meticulously, SRs are not always appropriate foundations for health care decisions (Malterud et al., 2016a). Sometimes, when the appraisal of the individual primary studies concludes that their quality is acceptable, the overall quality of documentation is not necessarily sufficient for the study's purpose. For example, we might imagine that a cohort study of good quality would offer better evidence than a weak RCT, even when the question deals with the effects of an intervention (Shaneyfelt, 2016).

A relevant response from the Cochrane Collaboration to such objections was that SRs should also include a standardized appraisal of the quality of evidence for each conclusion and reflections about the degree of confidence in the SR's recommendations. For this purpose, the Grading of Recommendations Assessment, Development and Evaluation working group developed *GRADE* (Guyatt et al., 2008). The GRADE system can also be used to evaluate the balance between benefits and adverse effects. GRADE includes an evaluation of the *risk of bias* of incoming evidence according to a checklist developed by Cochrane (Higgins & Green, 2011). By asking questions about randomization and blinding, this methodology is well suited to evaluate RCTs but is of no use for qualitative primary studies.

GRADE is not intended to be a checklist that assesses overall quality of the SR but a declaration of the strength and contents of outgoing evidence and recommendations, with a systematic appraisal of incoming evidence as the point of reference. NOKC always finishes its systematic reviews with grading according to these principles. Appraisal includes study design, study quality, consistency, directness, precision and publication bias for studies from which the data for each outcome measure were drawn. The grading of how much we may trust the certainty of evidence is presented as follows (Guyatt et al., 2008):

- *High quality* – Further research is very unlikely to change our confidence in the estimate of effect.
- *Moderate quality* – Further research is likely to have an important impact on our confidence in the estimate of effect and may change the estimate.
- *Low quality* – Further research is very likely to have an important impact on our confidence in the estimate of effect and is likely to change the estimate.
- *Very low quality* – Any estimate of effect is very uncertain.

New pyramids

The first evidence pyramid from Dartmouth and Yale illustrated the hierarchy for designs of primary studies as the basis for decisions about interventions and policy. Later, the Cochrane environment developed and promoted new pyramids, drawing attention and attributing priority to summarized research evidence that was available and elaborated for practical implementation. At the bottom of the pyramids, we find peer-reviewed individual studies with methodology not explicitly specified, then synopses of individual studies summing up evidence and synthesis as the next level up. The new hierarchies prioritize synopsis and especially synthesis rather than primary studies, while the original idea of RCTs as the ultimate methodology now seems to be more or less taken for granted. At the top of the prevailing evidence pyramids, we find systems where the new SRs have been implemented in guidelines with accompanying digital tools for practical use (see Figure 4.2). In searching for the best evidence, we start from the top and work our way down, whether we are clinicians, researchers or policymakers.

In principle, these new pyramids also may include qualitative primary studies and metasyntheses, although any such reference is only implicit. The new evidence hierarchies communicate the message that the quality of outgoing evidence is best when it can be transformed into standardized guidelines. For research knowledge in general, however, this is not a valid operationalization of evidence quality, even

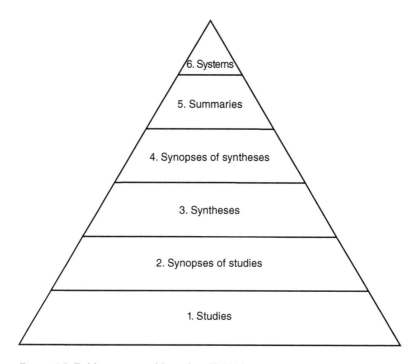

Figure 4.2 Evidence pyramid version 6S 2016.
Source: Adapted from (Alper & Haynes, 2016, p. 123). Redrawn from 6S pyramid for finding preappraised evidence, Brian S Apler and R Brian Haynes, EBHC pyramid 5.0 for accessing preappraised evidence and guidance, *Evid Based Med* 10.1136/ ebmed-2016-110447, 2016.

when we assume that qualitative evidence should lead to implementation and be transformed into better practice.

For evidence from qualitative primary studies and qualitative meta-syntheses, new insights and individualized practices may be a more adequate purpose, even though they are more difficult to specify and document (Popay et al., 1998; Malterud, 2001a; Thorne, 2017). From a clinical perspective, synthesis of knowledge about experiences and meanings of individuals' lives and health is a very different mission than standardized evidence developed to support policymaking (Malterud, 2019).

Diversity or standardization of knowledge

Variation and subjectivity are vital elements of qualitative studies. Taking this as a starting point, we explore and interpret experiences and meaning in context. We emphasize diversity and breadth to understand the particular, not to discover the universal. Quantitative meta-analysis, on the other hand, implies a standardization of definitions and procedures, with representativity and reproducibility as conditions for generalizability. When using qualitative metasynthesis as a research method, we need to recognize such epistemological oppositions, especially when appraising the sustainability of the evidence.

Merging apples and oranges – the synthesis of heterogeneous data

When working with a qualitative metasynthesis, you will notice that the primary studies that provide empirical data in the format of results are very *heterogeneous*. A recurring question about qualitative metasynthesis is whether it is at all possible to synthesize research findings of such mixed character (Dixon-Woods et al., 2005). Is it methodologically acceptable to merge apples and oranges (Gough & Thomas, 2017)?

This may be applied to synthesis of studies with different philosophical assumptions, such as phenomenology and Grounded theory. Furthermore, the research questions across the primary studies will only be identical in exceptional cases, meaning that the two authors or sets of authors did not study precisely the same phenomenon. Data collection using different methods, such as individual interviews and participant observations, may offer access to knowledge of very different kinds. Several methods for analysis are applied and reported with vastly different levels of details and accuracy. In studies with an explicitly theoretical frame of reference, the authors will approach different aspects of the phenomenon under study. Last but not least, the results from different qualitative studies are reported in very different textual formats.

Some of these variations indicate that qualitative research methods are not always used and presented with a sufficient degree of reflexivity and intersubjectivity. It may simply be difficult to recognize what has been done, what has been found and the impact of those findings. More often, however, diversity and variation are not merely legitimate - they are actually positive. In qualitative metasynthesis, heterogeneity that is not a reflection of inferior scholarship can inspire us in synthesis and upcycling (Thorne, 2017). I support Paterson (2001), who calls attention to a pragmatic standpoint regarding a diversity of qualitative methods among the primary studies.

To extend the metaphor of apples and oranges, we might argue that since both are fruits, metasynthesis may offer the opportunity to make a fruit salad with different though related ingredients, where the flavours of the apples and the oranges combine to create a new and even better taste. We must balance the ingredients so that one does not overwhelm the other while taking care that the pieces of fruit salad do not become so small that we lose all sense of the original flavours.

Robust organization of the literature review and the empirical data can prevent chaos in the research process. With the common epistemological basis of the primary studies in the interpretative paradigm (see above), reflexivity may contribute to analytic strategies in which diversity is valued and does not disturb the reader. Let us therefore use the opportunities presented by qualitative methods to develop evidence that either cannot or will not be standardized (Malterud, 2019). At the same time, we must be alert to where lines are crossed – which kinds of diversity are manageable in qualitative metasynthesis in an analytic and scholarly manner, and when do we simply have to realize that this is becoming too difficult?

Sustainable evidence

A great deal of the methodology for systematic and transparent searches and reviews of literature developed within the EBM tradition is also useful for qualitative metasynthesis (Gough et al., 2017b; Malterud, 2019). Still, several researchers have pointed out that even when this methodology is specifically adapted to qualitative metasynthesis, the distinctive footprints of quantitative logic may lead to inappropriate oversimplification (Petticrew, 2015; Thorne, 2017). Booth (2016) demonstrates how generic standards established for SRs in the Cochrane tradition are not universally appropriate. Checklists and quality criteria that are not specifically elaborated for qualitative metasynthesis may therefore be completely misleading when used for that kind of study. This point becomes especially clear when we discuss the sustainability of the evidence, especially if we apply traditional criteria from the positivist paradigm, such as generalizability and repeatability (Popay et al., 1998; Saini & Shlonsky, 2012; Malterud, 2019).

Transferability is an important criterion for qualitative studies, with the evidence in some way or another expected to provide new insights in contexts beyond the one in which the study was conducted (Malterud, 2001b). Transferability is closely connected to context, and evidence from qualitative studies may be regarded as situated knowledges (Haraway, 1991) (see above). No evidence is universally transferable or sustainable – it depends on the purpose of applying the knowledge and which questions are supposed to be answered by means of such knowledge. This is why qualitative metasynthesis should never claim *generalizability* (Malterud, 2019). My own recommendation is to establish and remain in a continuous dialogue with the practice domain, encouraging analysis directed by questions of relevance which can offer surprises, new understanding and have an impact on practice.

Still, results from this type of literature reviews do deserve conscientious reflections about transferability to individuals, population groups and related situations. This is especially important when the evidence is used as the foundation of decisions in health care. Several SRs deal with the effects of complex interventions. It may be difficult to draw sustainable conclusions – independent of topic and research question – from the standardized methodology inherent in this format, and many researchers agree that it is not suited to answer any and all kinds of questions (Greenhalgh, 2012; Lewin et al., 2012; Ioannidis, 2016; Malterud et al., 2016a).

Qualitative evidence is knowledge about the particular and the subjective rather than the universal and the objective (McWhinney, 1989). The ontology of clinical practice therefore requires an epistemology where particulars and diversity are celebrated, explored and interpreted, even when uncertainty is the inevitable price to be paid (Malterud et al., 2017). An SR and the summing up of knowledge offering insights into and an understanding of the lives and health of individuals therefore has a different potential for transferability than standardized knowledge developed with generalizability on a population level as a core premise (Lewin et al., 2018). This does not, however, mean that the evidence is necessarily less sustainable. We will of course exercise caution when evidence from a qualitative metasynthesis is used for recommendations and guidelines that involve larger population groups. If ambitions of generalizability imply that we must renounce the hallmarks of qualitative methods, the sustainability of our evidence will suffer (Malterud, 2019).

Three steps forward and two steps back

Several authors recommend that strategies for data collection and analysis for SRs be determined in advance, that a study protocol only be amended for exceptional reasons and that criteria for the inclusion and exclusion of hits from the literature search be determined ahead of time (Popay et al., 1998; Liberati et al., 2009; Nasjonalt kunnskapssenter for helsetjenesten, 2015).

Consequently, we might imagine that some of the challenges presented above could be resolved by standardizing the knowledge base. An ethnographic study of the methodology for SRs demonstrates how standardization may contribute to reducing the connection to the original aim of the study (Moreira, 2007). It can also be argued that this kind of standardization cuts off the input from important sources of critical reflection. However, it is also a matter of current debate whether the actual principles actually ensure sufficiently sustainable evidence also for quantitative SRs and meta-analyses (Ioannidis, 2016).

In a qualitative study, the course of action is normally adjusted along the way, based on learning and insights from experiences and the data, so that the study's focus is sharpened. Similar approaches will also enhance the sustainability of a qualitative metasynthesis. *Iteration* implies that something is repeated several times to achieve a certain goal, but even with flexibility and motion as necessary preconditions for an iterative strategy, a casual and muddy procedure is still not legitimate. It is vital to keep one's head while remaining accessible to re-evaluation of one's strategies. The decision trail will help us maintain an overview that will allow us to recapitulate how and why certain choices were made. These are legitimate aspects of qualitative research, implying, for example, that data collection and analysis should walk hand in hand as a stepwise process (Popay et al., 1998). These principles are most systematically promoted in Grounded theory with the analytical strategy of constant comparison (Glaser & Strauss, 1967).

Iterative strategies imply that we will often go three steps forward and two steps back, with the insights obtained *en route* helping to develop the analysis. Several authors consider *flexibility* and *dependability* to be basic premises of a qualitative method (Hamberg et al., 1994). With qualitative metasynthesis, we will also seize the opportunity provided by the increased understanding obtained by learning from experiences along the way. Flexibility is important in the process of sampling, where the inclusion of primary studies from the literature search should be adjusted if that would help strengthen the information power and support the sustainability of the incoming evidence. During analysis, it is also essential that we do not blindly follow a predetermined path but remain open to revising our research question little by little.

In any case, the process must be systematic and transparent. Intersubjectivity, meaning that we give the reader access to the path we followed, is more important than trying to ensure that the reader would have chosen exactly the same path (Malterud, 1993). In practice, this may imply that we invest time in developing a robust research protocol and adjusting the research question, search strategy and ongoing analysis as far as is necessary, while we document the process, explain our choices and invite the reader to grasp the systematics that we have followed.

Grading of qualitative metasynthesis

The SR methodology was established as a tool for evidence-based policy and practice in health care. The GRADE system (see above) was developed to grade the confidence of the evidence base, but the outgoing evidence was still not always relevant for the purpose and context of the application, even if acceptable grades were obtained. Questions about feasibility, acceptability and local preconditions were also essential to assess the results of interventions (Lewin et al., 2012). Gradually, the need for systematic grading of evidence from qualitative studies emerged when such reviews were intended to serve as the basis for decision-making.

In 2010, the World Health Organization established a panel to prepare guidelines that would optimize health worker roles in improving access to key maternal and new-born health interventions through task shifting (World Health Organization). Evidence from qualitative metasyntheses was emphasized (Glenton et al., 2013), leading to the development of the *GRADE-CERQual* (Confidence in the evidence from reviews of qualitative research) (Lewin et al., 2015; Glenton et al., 2016b). CERQual is an element of the GRADE system and is based on GRADE principles, while still intended to adhere to the methodological principles of qualitative research.

The method includes a structured assessment of four components (Lewin et al., 2015):

1   Methodological limitations
2   Relevance
3   Coherence
4   Adequacy of data

Each component is graded in levels as high, moderate, low or very low. CERQual is not intended to be a tool for the general quality assessment of qualitative metasyntheses – rather, it has been developed to support people using findings from qualitative evidence synthesis in decision-making processes and guidelines (Lewin et al., 2015, 2018). In other words, the sustainability of outgoing evidence for the various findings in a qualitative metasynthesis is judged according to the incoming evidence. Confidence in evidence depends on the extent to which a review finding is a reasonable representation of the phenomenon under study (Lewin et al., 2018).

Like GRADE, CERQual reassesses appraisals that have already been conducted regarding relevance, methodological quality and empirical data during the preparation of the SR and the synthesis. It differs in deliberately emphasizing the role of the individual primary studies for outgoing evidence. Furthermore, *coherence* between the results of the primary studies and the results from the synthesis is evaluated: how clear and cogent is the fit between the data from the primary studies and a review finding that synthesizes that data (Colvin et al., 2018)? Deviating data from the primary studies may, according to CERQual, indicate that the primary studies are not sufficiently rich and complex, that deviating findings have been insufficiently explored or that the sample did not have sufficient information power. When such variations are difficult to explain, coherence is rated as less convincing, and less confidence is attributed to the evidence (Colvin et al., 2018).

It is easy to approve the CERQual contributors' intentions to try to improve the reporting of qualitative primary studies and the systematic evaluation of outgoing evidence from qualitative metasyntheses. On the other hand, unequivocality and coherence are not appropriate standards for qualitative studies – indeed, the opposite may be true. Furthermore, policy making is often not the purpose of qualitative research. Using these research methods, we pursue different nuances and aspects of the phenomena we study, especially when analysis is more on the interpretative than on the descriptive side, as with metasynthesis. Surprises and paradoxes are regarded as valuable indications of diversity, not as signs of the low sustainability of incoming evidence. Contradictions and discomfort may characterize qualitative evidence of appropriate and nuanced quality. It is just these kinds of variations that will determine whether we can develop new knowledge and not simply reproduce what we already knew (Wong, 2016). Therefore, not every result will fit into any context, and discrepancies, incoherence and ambiguity within the results are natural and even desirable as an added benefit of interpretation.

This is why it is problematic when low confidence is assigned to findings from one primary study which are not coherent with findings from the other primary studies. Critical reflection on the sustainability of incoming and outgoing evidence is important in qualitative metasynthesis, but it is questionable whether it can ever be standardized without essential elements being lost. Therefore, we can ask with good reason how far it is possible to synthesize studies with situated and contextually dependent incoming evidence and to what degree outgoing evidence actually should and can be transformed into recommendations and guidelines (Lewin et al., 2018; Malterud, 2019).

One important finding from Fosse's metasynthesis about the role of the NHD at the end of life (2014) was how complicated it could be when the next of kin, who were supposed to take vital decisions on the patient's behalf, did not have sufficient knowledge about the patient's preferences.

Similarly, different primary studies demonstrated that a doctor and patient might have diametrically opposed understandings of the causes of CFS/ME (Larun & Malterud, 2007). These kinds of contradictions cannot be emphasized when the methodological pivot assumes rigid coherence. Noblit and Hare (1988) call particular attention to the impact of such perspectives in what they call refutational synthesis (see Chapter 3), and Dixon-Woods (2005) warns against strategies for analysis that only reproduce and sum up the commonalities of previous research.

With the criterion of coherence, the CERQual method communicates standards of unambiguous and standardized bases for decision-making as possible and desirable, a standpoint that many stakeholders would welcome. Still, I am not sure that this will be an adequate point of departure for grading qualitative metasyntheses, in which the aim is to highlight the particular rather than the universal. CERQual is, however, under continuous development, and the final version has not yet been written.

Mixed methods and qualitative metasynthesis

A *mixed methods* (MM) design implies that the researcher uses more than one research method in a single study. With the synthesis of the different types of results developed from different positions, a *multi-methodological* study may offer a basis for broader insight and more nuances. The focus for this book is qualitative metasynthesis, and the aim is neither to cover all kinds of SRs nor to provide a comprehensive presentation of MMs. In the literature search of a qualitative metasynthesis, however, we often encounter primary studies with different designs that must be evaluated for inclusion. Based on my experience, these situations often give rise to certain methodological considerations that are briefly discussed below.

Qualitative and quantitative methods in the same study

Most often, the term MM is used to denote multi-methodological studies in which qualitative and quantitative research methods are combined, with the results integrated in a synthesis (Creswell & Clark, 2011). Projects integrating findings from sub-studies with different quantitative or qualitative methods are also called MM studies, even though this combination is not very common. The MM approach may be understood as a kind of *triangulation*, although with a higher analytic level of ambition than when different studies are simply juxtaposed (Migiro & Magangi, 2011).

Results from the different studies may concur, contradict or expand on one another (Östlund et al., 2011). With analysis, the findings from the different methodological approaches are assumed to complement one another and to shed light on different dimensions but not to compete about what is most "true" (Teddlie & Tashakkori, 2009). A vital precondition is that the synthesis is conducted so that the findings from the different approaches are integrated with due respect for their methodological distinctions.

An example of an MM study combining qualitative and quantitative methods is Larun's PhD thesis «Kronisk utmattelsessyndrom. Kunnskap, aktivitet og utfordringer» [English: CFS: Knowledge, activity and challenges] (2011), which draws on two SRs (one qualitative, one quantitative) and a focus group study. The main findings from these three studies are summed up, synthesized and discussed in a compelling way, supported by relevant theoretical perspectives.

Multi-methodological exploration of complex research questions

There are good arguments that SRs need to be complemented with qualitative studies to understand the context and preconditions for interventions to be explored or implemented in health care (Mays et al., 2005; Wong, 2016). MM studies are therefore often promoted as a response to the critique of research with traditional effect studies that offer only limited and simplified knowledge about complex research questions and systems (Oxman et al., 2010/2014; Campbell-Scherer, 2012; Glenton et al., 2013; Shaw, 2015).

Analogous critiques, although reversed, may be raised against qualitative metasynthesis, depending on the research question. This is one of several reasons to be interested in how knowledge developed from different ontological and epistemological assumptions may communicate in the best way and contribute to more diversity in our knowledge capital. Another point to be considered is deciding on what role potential primary MM studies are to be assigned in the sample of a qualitative metasynthesis.

Qualitative metasynthesis with mixed methods

The literature search of a qualitative metasynthesis will often dig up some primary studies with MM designs. In her study about the role of the NHD at the end of life, Fosse identified a survey in which 49% of the participants (N = 104) responded to an open-ended question at the end of the questionnaire that asked what else might be important for care at the end of life (Vohra et al., 2006). As with all other candidate studies, such studies must be appraised for relevance and quality, and Fosse concluded that this one complied with the inclusion criteria.

Often, however, an MM study must be excluded, even when its research question at first seems relevant to the metasynthesis (Atkins et al., 2008). This may occur, for example, when evidence from one of the paradigms is given priority, while evidence from the other paradigm is used in a non-committal fashion. In other cases, the presentation of the method or results from this kind of study may lack the transparency needed to identify which results originate from which data sources.

The MM design was developed for empirical primary studies combining qualitative and quantitative methods. Several authors have also presented metasynthesis methods that include both qualitative and quantitative primary studies, such as Dixon-Woods et al. with Critical interpretive synthesis (2006) and Pawson et al. with Realist synthesis (2005) (see Chapter 3).

Such approaches may be called *MM metasyntheses*. On the basis of a literature search with 17,962 hits, Tricco et al. identified 121 studies where methods for the integration of qualitative and quantitative data were discussed or used (Tricco et al., 2016). Seven different such methods for MM metasynthesis were identified. The authors evaluated the similarities and differences, and strengths and weaknesses in these methods, concluding that, although the results were often presented with rich, contextually based data, specific descriptions of the analytic method were lacking in most cases.

A significant amount of methodological development is needed before MM metasyntheses can provide sufficiently sustainable evidence. Still, there are examples suggesting that this may be an achievable goal. Munthe-Kaas et al. (2013) published an SR about the effects and experiences of interventions to promote continuity in residential child care institutions and influence the psychosocial development of the children they serve. The review summarizes and integrates the results from six effect studies about different interventions with results from nine qualitative studies about the experiences of clients regarding the included interventions. The outcome, especially from the qualitative studies, documents a wish for stability and structure, predictability, attachment to and availability of fewer caregivers and a clear preference for the continuity that comes from the cohabitation model.

When carrying out a unifying and committed synthesis of data developed from different paradigms, it is necessary to be aware of and find acceptable compromises for the epistemological challenges that arise. Today, I find this to be an arduous strategy that would not be my first choice for metasynthesis. A less complicated alternative for reviews of research including both qualitative and quantitative studies is to recapitulate the main findings as a narrative review, without aspiring to more ambitious analysis and synthesis (see Chapter 1). In this case, we leave the idea of metasynthesis in the format I have chosen to define and present in this book.

Synthesis of qualitative primary studies with different designs

Studies blending different quantitative methods, such as a cross-sectional study and an RCT, are sometimes also called MM studies. Similar terminology might also be used to denote studies where the researchers used different types of qualitative methods, such as participant observation and focus group interviews, although this is not so common. These kinds of studies have many similarities with qualitative metasynthesis, where the included primary studies are usually very heterogeneous in terms of data collection and analysis. Normally, our sample will contain articles characterized by very different extents and types of theoretical commitment and a variety of methodological traditions.

My own experience is that the synthesis and upcycling of different types of qualitative studies creates a lot of methodological challenges. Still, I find these challenges to be manageable and fundamentally different from what I have discussed above regarding MM synthesis, which strives to integrate qualitative and quantitative studies. There may indeed be considerable variations in the principles, conduct and presentation of different qualitative studies. Still, this kind of variety reminds me of the diversity which is an inherent element of a focus group study, with participants being very different as to experiences and communicative power, and of interviews conducted with different moderators taking a variety of routes, although the point of departure is similar. At the end of the day, these studies share certain crucial epistemological assumptions regarding sample, analysis, interpretation and transferability.

In the metasynthesis about CFS/ME experiences, primary studies based on individual interviews, group interviews and observational studies together offered a broad picture with many relevant nuances (Larun & Malterud, 2007). In the metasynthesis about experiences among lesbian families encountering the maternity ward, most primary studies were interview studies that used phenomenological or thematic analysis (Dahl et al., 2013). First, we almost always find some common themes across the dissimilarities. Second, this kind of diversity of data may offer an unexpected bonus by giving access to nuances and contradictions that we did not have the imagination to actively seek out (Thorne, 2017).

5   Final comments

Ethics and privacy protection

Research in medicine and health care is obliged to take heed of issues related to ethics and confidentiality. In most high-income countries, such issues are regulated by laws and regulations intended to guarantee that the interests related to the participants' welfare and integrity is given priority before interests related to science and society. This body of rules has been designed to ensure individuals' security and informed consent. In conducting a qualitative metasynthesis, we are also expected to follow these regulations for research ethics, even though some adjustment is needed. It is therefore essential to acknowledge the intentions of these rules.

Regulations and approvals

The Helsinki Declaration was first presented in 1964, primarily to protect patients as participants in experimental research. Since then, extensive revisions have been undertaken (World Medical Association, 2013). The declaration represents international consensus about medical research ethics and deals, among other items, with interventions associated with risks or burdens, research on vulnerable groups, protocols, informed consent, the use of placebos and publication of the research results.

The Helsinki Declaration also formed the basis for establishing *committees for medical and health research ethics*. The precise arrangements are different in different countries. Health research in Norway or in the UK, for example, requires approval from Research Ethics Committees, who ask questions about participant consent, participant and researcher safety, protection of the rights of vulnerable persons and data protection.

Whilst ethics bodies differ across countries, in projects where qualitative metasynthesis is used as method, approval from such a body would not usually be necessary. Nevertheless, a proper judgment of such issues entails knowledge of the regulations affecting the primary studies. It would also be useful to attend to guidance and checklists for the evaluation of research ethics prepared by the national committees for medical and health research ethics, see for example information from UK and Canada (Government of Canada; National Institute for Health Research).

When conducting qualitative metasyntheses, we do not have direct contact with patients. We use neither personal archives nor individually recognizable data and it is difficult to imagine how this design would represent any risk for individuals who participated in the primary studies. We must also assume that the authors of the primary studies that we include for analysis have obtained the necessary approvals. Such issues are, however, not always sufficiently clearly stated in the articles presenting the primary studies. In a metasynthesis about lesbian families encountering the maternity ward, Dahl explored how matters of research ethics had been presented (Dahl, 2015). Among the 13 primary studies included for analysis, nine had explicit information about ethical evaluation and approval. All 13 studies were still included, though special attention was given to how quotations were used in the metasynthesis.

Distance as a challenge

Medical research ethics also reflect general ethical norms. Vetlesen (1994) discusses individuals' preconditions for *moral behaviour* and says that empathy is necessary to assess whether a situation is *morally significant*. The foundations of moral behaviour are insight, judgment and action. Vetlesen argues that proximity is a critical precondition to recognize another person as a *moral addressee*, someone who will be affected by one's moral behaviour.

As researchers in qualitative primary studies, we usually meet face to face with the participants. In that context, we will seldom forget that the participants are our moral addressees. In conducting a qualitative metasynthesis, however, the authors have no contact with the participants from the primary studies or, usually, the researchers who initially collected and analysed the data from these participants (Campbell et al., 2011). We take for granted that the participants gave informed consent. We do not have to ask the researchers to elaborate evidence from articles that are already published. No efforts are needed to establish trust and secure confidentiality. In Fosse's metasynthesis about the role of the nursing home doctor (NHD) at the end of life (2014), two of the primary studies had been conducted in Scandinavia, with the others from USA and Canada, where the material and cultural conditions for health and illness are very different from those found in Norway. When the distance between the actors involved in a research project becomes that large, we may easily forget the anonymous participants and the named researchers as moral addressees to whom we must pay due respect during our work.

In qualitative studies, with interpretation as our strategy for the development of knowledge, we have an ethical obligation to ensure that what is said and written will not be misunderstood or distorted. Such issues are related to the internal validity of the study but also involve the trust the participants have shown by sharing their experiences and knowledge. *Dialogic validation* is often used in a qualitative primary study, with the researcher checking with the participant that a given message has been perceived in roughly the way it was meant. Qualitative metasynthesis does not offer this opportunity to either researcher or participant. In these studies, we are obliged to accept the primary study authors' interpretations as the point of departure for our own interpretations. Many important nuances may get lost during the process by which existing evidence is upcycled in our analysis and synthesis. We may show the participants and the authors of the primary studies respect by being sensitive as to how we sum up what they thought and meant and how we take care of quotations that may come from a completely different context.

It may be tempting to draw extensive conclusions about lifeworld and content of meaning when we have numerous rich and relevant results to sum up, especially when there is a large distance in time and space from those who shared their perspectives and from the researchers who first presented the results. Take care not to jump to conclusions! We should be reminded that we not only have a methodological responsibility to consider the meaning but also an ethical obligation to evaluate the limitations and sustainability of what we can safely conclude. During the research process, we could take the time to imagine the human beings who contributed to the knowledge we want to synthesize. In this way, the distance between metasynthesis researcher and original study participant may somehow become reduced.

Contributing something new

Qualitative studies are supposed to develop and present new knowledge. For primary studies, this means an obligation with regard to the participants. We abuse their trust and waste their time if our research simply repeats what is already known. Analogous considerations may be valid with metasynthesis regarding our analytic ambitions – we intend to conduct a synthesis revealing something more and something else than the primary studies that we have included. Being researchers, we have a responsibility towards those who fund our study, in addition to a responsibility towards the society of science and the practice domain. Screening endless lists of publications identified by impetuously searches is not always compliant with ethical conduct. It may also be an important aim to contribute to better health or health care for the patient or population group that the project deals with, especially if it is a vulnerable group (Bondas & Hall, 2007a), not only sorting and reiterating a big pile of references.

The researcher should therefore not simply create a puzzle for his or her entertainment but prepare the design and methodology plans so that the results may become sustainable deposits in the scientific bank of knowledge (Malterud, 2019). In this way, there is also an ethical obligation to stretch as much as possible when it comes to using the synthesis to develop knowledge that may make a difference for somebody (Stige et al., 2009).

What do you need to conduct a qualitative metasynthesis?

In research, the aim of the study will always determine the kind of method that will provide the best answers. Our strategies for recruitment and data collection will have an impact on the kind of data we have available for elaboration and analysis. Our methodological skills will have a strong influence on how we succeed in planning, preparing and conducting our project. Editors and peer reviewers evaluate whether our findings merit publication and a wider audience. What, then, is especially important to reflect on when you consider whether qualitative metasynthesis will become the path you choose for your project?

Competence and experience

Qualitative metasynthesis is one of several qualitative research methods and entails the appraisal of many different designs. You will therefore need more than basic knowledge of and skills in the principles and procedures for qualitative research. Ideally, you will have some methodological breadth. Without such qualifications, you will be challenged to understand the vital assumptions underlying the research process, especially regarding appraisal, extraction, analysis, interpretation and synthesis of data. For qualitative metasynthesis, it is not enough to have extensive experience in other types of research – on the contrary, this may contribute to a position where you are not able to assess your own methodological limitations in a sufficiently critical manner. Previous experiences from other types of SRs can be useful resources but are not necessary preconditions. In my experience, the skills required for this part of the process are not terribly challenging to acquire. Methodological reflection is still important.

It is a great advantage if you have hands-on experience with qualitative analysis from one or more empirical primary studies. If you have not conducted a similar research process to those presented by the authors of the primary studies you include in your metasynthesis, it may be difficult for you to imagine and understand the strategies, challenges, choices and compromises underlying the results on which you are going to elaborate (Thorne, 2017). I do not think the specific kind of qualitative method you have experienced is of great importance – your most important resources are your previous encounters with the research process itself. You should nevertheless take all the time needed to familiarize yourself with the specific method you choose for your metasynthesis.

If neither you nor your supervisors or collaborators have had any such experiences, I recommend that you instead start by preparing for an empirical primary study to explore your topic. In that case, you can take advantage of your interest to obtain an overview of the research literature by conducting a thorough literature search as part of your project preparations, in order to prevent research waste (Chalmers et al., 2014) and strengthen your opportunities to publish new knowledge. Then, you may also better consider whether your research question is best studied with a qualitative or a quantitative method.

Relevant primary studies with useful presentations of results

You might use qualitative metasynthesis as a strategy to look into a topic for which you know – or at least believe – limited research is available. At a minimum, you want to check thoroughly for what there is, and it may be tempting to try to sum it up. You might find that there is not much to summarize. Even when you start the process with a literature search that produces a large number of hits, you may realize that only a few articles have sufficient relevance, quality and sustainability for synthesis. Even if you think that you have just enough material to proceed, you may later discover that the presentations of results from the primary studies you include are actually meagre or unclear and that rich descriptions and interpretations are rare in your sample (Geertz, 2000).

Noblit and Hare (1988) recommend that you undertake a painstaking evaluation of such issues before you set out on analysis and synthesis and that you terminate the project if you do not have sufficiently sustainable data as incoming evidence. There might be several quantitative but few qualitative studies about your topic. If so, you might use that as motivation to conduct an empirical primary study with a qualitative research method. It is, however, also possible that your literature search has not been sufficiently accurate and that it is worth the effort to try again with new search terms and more or different bibliographic sources.

Resources and personal traits

In my experience, undertaking a qualitative metasynthesis makes professional library competence and assistance absolutely essential. You may certainly plan, prepare and conduct a search on your own, but it is difficult for a layperson (in library terms) to do this in a reflexive and systematic way that can later be documented, and in these kinds of studies, such documentation is expected. If these resources are not available, you should either try to establish a collaboration with a library or choose another approach to your research question.

Some personal traits may also play a role when considering qualitative metasynthesis as your potential method. A systematic and transparent procedure is especially important with this method. If you do not have the personal capacity to work in a tidy and highly organized fashion, you may easily end up in chaos, surrounded by an enormous number of seemingly impenetrable references. In this kind of study, you can be sure that there will always be much to keep track of. You may complement your talents of this kind by establishing good systems and using all available tools. Advice about such things is probably available from a colleague with practical experience.

As a researcher undertaking a qualitative metasynthesis, you will encounter a broad diversity of primary studies. Some of their authors may have used other procedures and chosen other perspectives than you would have. Several authors emphasize the importance of approaching the field with an open and undogmatic spirit, because you will have to accept several kinds of pragmatic compromises along the way (Sandelowski, 2012; Thorne, 2017).

Set off!

Qualitative metasynthesis is one out of many available strategies for upcycling research evidence, developing the research field and strengthening our knowledge capital. You stand on the shoulders of your predecessors and use their products as your platform for further efforts. In this way, you can join in building something together, rather than sowing a seed in your own way. This book may serve as your map, but you must also be prepared to take your own decisions, make the compromises you feel are needed and defend those decisions.

You are not alone

You may have already conducted a focus group study as the first sub-project of your PhD. Because you worked hard on recruitment, you were able to include participants with a broad range of experience and collected data of appropriate information power. Collaborating with your supervisor, you learned the skills for managing and analysing qualitative data, and a colleague provided useful suggestions regarding theoretical perspectives that made it easier for you to write a concise article. At the end of the writing phase, however, you realize that there was already quite a lot of research literature about your topic that you did not see on the radar during your initial literature searches. You admit that you need to establish a better overview of the area and consider doing a new, comprehensive search before you proceed with the interview study you have planned as your second sub-project.

Newer and more exciting

You make an appointment with the research librarian to sort out how best to proceed. In discussions about aims, search terms and databases, you find out that the terminology for your topic is not as clear and consistent as you had thought. This discovery helps explain why several references and authors now pop up as new acquaintances, and you even stumble upon a couple of articles that seem to be nearly identical with the upcoming sub-study you have planned. A test search results in large amounts of contamination, but you also see exciting references that you look forward to engaging with. It turns out that there are already several qualitative studies on the topic. The librarian offers to assist you in preparing an SR and, after discussions with your supervisor, you decide to concentrate on an identification, analysis and synthesis of relevant qualitative studies.

Wheat or chaff?

Together, you will revise the research question, adjust the search strategy and try to balance sensitivity and specificity in a feasible fashion to sharpen the output and reduce the contamination. Some first-class primary studies that you found by accident offer some interesting concepts that will strengthen your search. You wonder how it is possible to get at so many articles that are far beyond your subject of interest, but fortunately, you notice that there is also some promising material. It may be tempting to let yourself become absorbed in technical details, but you are still able to organize your screening of the hits from the literature search without any chaos or much duplication of effort. You start in on the analysis and synthesis of the results from the 14 primary studies included as your data, and you realize that it is only now that the research process is really underway. Every article is not equally excellent, but you still learn many new things related to your research question, both thematically and methodologically. You are tempted to familiarize yourself more with some of the authors.

Sustainable competence – new opportunities for collaboration

It turns out the analysis and writing were more taxing than you had expected. Still, you notice how much you can use of what you learnt during your first focus group study. Some of the primary studies guided you towards new and exciting theoretical perspectives that you become acquainted with, considering the possibilities of using them in a more committed manner to sharpen the presentation and discussion of your metasynthesis. Your supervisor has substantial experience in this kind of research and wants you to push yourself on your own as far as possible without giving you the feeling that you are completely alone in this work. Writing takes a great deal of time – much more than you thought – but after some rounds of peer reviews and revisions, your article is finally published. You present your research at a conference in Boston. It turns out that two people in the audience are authors of primary studies that you especially appreciated and used in this metasynthesis. Over lunch you talk more and discuss the possibilities of planning a new collaborative project.

References

Aase, M., Nordrehaug, J. E., & Malterud, K. (2008). "If you cannot tolerate that risk, you should never become a physician": A qualitative study about existential experiences among physicians. *J Med Ethics, 34*(11), 767–771. doi:10.1136/jme.2007.023275

Alper, B. S., & Haynes, R. B. (2016). EBHC pyramid 5.0 for accessing preappraised evidence and guidance. *Evid Based Med, 21*(4), 123–125. doi:10.1136/ebmed-2016-110447

Alvesson, M., & Sköldberg, K. (2009). *Reflexive methodology: New vistas for qualitative research* (2nd ed.). Los Angeles, CA and London: SAGE.

Anderson, V. R., Jason, L. A., Hlavaty, L. E., Porter, N., & Cudia, J. (2011). A review and meta-synthesis of qualitative studies on myalgic encephalomyelitis/chronic fatigue syndrome. *Patient Educ Couns*, 147–155. doi:10.1016/j.pec.2011.04.016

Arksey, H., & O'Malley, L. (2005). Scoping studies: Towards a methodological framework. *Int J Soc Res Meth, 8*(1), 19–32. doi:10.1080/1364557032000119616

Atkins, S., Lewin, S., Smith, H., Engel, M., Fretheim, A., & Volmink, J. (2008). Conducting a meta-ethnography of qualitative literature: Lessons learnt. *BMC Med Res Methodol, 8*, 21–. doi:10.1186/1471-2288-8-21

Atkinson, P., & Hammersley, M. (1994). Ethnography and participant observation. In N. K. Denzin & Y. S. Lincoln (Eds.), *Handbook of qualitative research* (pp. 248–261). Thousand Oaks, CA: SAGE.

Barnett-Page, E., & Thomas, J. (2009). Methods for the synthesis of qualitative research: A critical review. *BMC Med Res Methodol, 9*(1), 1–11. doi:10.1186/1471-2288-9-59

Biagioli, V., Piredda, M., Alvaro, R., & de Marinis, M. G. (2016). The experiences of protective isolation in patients undergoing bone marrow or haematopoietic stem cell transplantation: Systematic review and metasynthesis. *Eur J Cancer Care. Epub 2016/02/20.* doi:10.1111/ecc.12461

Black, N. (2001). Evidence based policy: Proceed with care. *BMJ, 323*(7307), 275–279.

Bondas, T., & Hall, E. O. (2007a). Challenges in approaching metasynthesis research. *Qual Health Res, 17*(1), 113–121. doi:10.1177/1049732306295879

Bondas, T., & Hall, E. O. C. (2007b). A decade of metasynthesis research in health sciences: A meta-method study. *Int J Qual Stud Health Well-being* *2*(2), 101–113. doi:10.1080/17482620701251684

Booth, A. (2016). Searching for qualitative research for inclusion in systematic reviews: A structured methodological review. *Syst Rev, 5*, 74. doi:10.1186/s13643-016-0249-x

Bousquet, G., Orri, M., Winterman, S., Brugiere, C., Verneuil, L., & Revah-Levy, A. (2015). Breaking bad news in oncology: A metasynthesis. *J Clin Oncol, 33*(22), 2437–2443. doi:10.1200/jco.2014.59.6759

Braun, V., & Clarke, V. (2006). Using thematic analysis in psychology. *Qual Res Psychol, 3*(2), 77–101. doi:10.1191/1478088706qp063oa

Britten, N., Campbell, R., Pope, C., Donovan, J., Morgan, M., & Pill, R. (2002). Using meta ethnography to synthesise qualitative research: A worked example. *J Health Serv Res Pol, 7*, 209–215. doi:10.1258/135581902320432732

Britten, N., Garside, R., Pope, C., Dip, J. F., & Cooper, C. (2017). Asking more of qualitative synthesis: A response to Sally Thorne. *Qual Health Res, 27*(9), 1370–1376. doi:10.1177/1049732317709010

Britten, N., & Pope, C. (2011). Medicine taking for asthma: A worked example of meta-ethnography. In K. Hannes & C. Lockwood (Eds.), *Synthesizing qualitative research.* (pp. 41–57). Chichester, England: John Wiley & Sons, Ltd.

Brown, I., Thompson, J., Tod, A., & Jones, G. (2006). Primary care support for tackling obesity: A qualitative study of the perceptions of obese patients. *Br J Gen Pract, 56*(530), 666–672.

Brunton, G., Stansfield, C., Caird, J., & Thomas, J. (2017). Finding relevant studies. In D. Gough, S. Oliver, & J. Thomas (Eds.), *An introduction to systematic reviews.*(2nd ed, pp. 93–122). London: SAGE.

Campbell, R., Pound, P., Morgan, M., Daker-White, G., Britten, N., Pill, R., et al. (2011). Evaluating meta-ethnography: Systematic analysis and synthesis of qualitative research. *Health Technol. Assess., 15*(43), 1–164.

Campbell, R., Pound, P., Pope, C., Britten, N., Pill, R., Morgan, M., et al. (2003). Evaluating meta-ethnography: A synthesis of qualitative research on lay experiences of diabetes and diabetes care. *Soc Sci Med, 56*, 671–684. doi:10.1016/s0277-9536(02)00064-3

Campbell-Scherer, D. (2012). The 11th hour–time for EBM to return to first principles? *Evid. Based Med., 17*(4), 103–104. doi:10.1136/ebmed-2012–100578

Canadian Task Force on the Periodic Health Examination. (1979). The periodic health examination. *Can Med Assoc. J, 121*(9), 1193–1254.

Carlsen, B., & Glenton, C. (2016). The swine flu vaccine, public attitudes, and researcher interpretations: A systematic review of qualitative research. *BMC Health Serv Res, 16*, 203. doi:10.1186/s12913-016-1466-7

Carlsen, B., Glenton, C., & Pope, C. (2007). Thou shalt versus thou shalt not: A meta-synthesis of GPs' attitudes to clinical practice guidelines. *Br J Gen Pract, 57*(545), 971–978.

Carroll, C., Booth, A., & Lloyd-Jones, M. (2012). Should we exclude inadequately reported studies from qualitative systematic reviews? An evaluation of sensitivity analyses in two case study reviews. *Qual Health Res, 22*, 1425–1434. doi:10.1177/1049732312452937

Centre for Reviews and Disssemination. (2008). *Systematic reviews. CRD's guidance for undertaking reviews in health care.* York: Centre for Reviews and Dissemination, University of York. http://www.york.ac.uk/inst/crd/pdf/Systematic_Reviews.pdf (20.12.2016).

Chalmers, I. (1993). The Cochrane Collaboration: Preparing, maintaining, and disseminating systematic reviews of the effects of health care. *Ann N Y Acad Sci, 703*, 156–163; discussion 163–155.

Chalmers, I., Bracken, M. B., Djulbegovic, B., Garattini, S., Grant, J., Gülmezoglu, A. M., et al. (2014). How to increase value and reduce waste when research priorities are set. *The Lancet, 383*(9912), 156–165. doi:10.1016/S0140-6736(13)62229-1

Chamberlain, K. (2000). Methodolatry and qualitative health research. *J Health Psychol, 5*(3), 285–296. doi:10.1177/135910530000500306

Christensen, M. E., Brincks, J., Schnieber, A., & Soerensen, D. (2016). The intention to exercise and the execution of exercise among persons with multiple sclerosis – A qualitative metasynthesis. *Disabil Rehabil, 38*(11), 1023–1033. doi:10.3109/09638288.2015.1091859

Cochrane, A. L. (1989). Archie Cochrane in his own words. Selections arranged from his 1972 introduction to "effectiveness and efficiency: Random reflections on the health services" 1972. *Control Clin Trials, 10*(4), 428–433.

Cochrane Collaboration. (2011). *Cochrane handbook for systematic reviews of interventions: 5.1.0 ed.* http://handbook.Cochrane.Org/ (15.03.2017).

Colquhoun, H. L., Levac, D., O'Brien, K. K., Straus, S., Tricco, A. C., Perrier, L., et al. (2014). Scoping reviews: Time for clarity in definition, methods, and reporting. *J Clin Epidemio., 67*(12), 1291–1294. doi:10.1016/j.jclinepi.2014.03.013

Colvin, C. J., Garside, R., Wainwright, M., Munthe-Kaas, H., Glenton, C., Bohren, M. A., et al. (2018). Applying grade-cerqual to qualitative evidence synthesis findings-paper 4: How to assess coherence. *Implement Sci: IS, 13*(Suppl 1), 13. doi:10.1186/s13012-017-0691-8s

Cooke, A., Smith, D., & Booth, A. (2012). Beyond PICO: The spider tool for qualitative evidence synthesis. *Qual Health Res, 22*(10), 1435–1443. doi:10.1177/1049732312452938

Cooper, I. D. (2016). What is a "mapping study?". *J Med Library Assoc, 104*(1), 76–78. doi:10.3163/1536-5050.104.1.013

Creswell, J. W. (2013). *Qualitative inquiry & research design: Choosing among five approaches* (3rd ed.). Los Angeles, CA: SAGE.

Creswell, J. W., & Clark, V. L. P. (2011). *Designing and conducting mixed methods research.* Los Angeles, CA: SAGE.

Critical Appraisal Skills Programme (CASP). (2013). *Qualitative research checklist.* http://media.Wix.Com/ugd/dded87_29c5b002d99342f788c6ac670e49f274.Pdf (04.08.2016).

Crotty, M. (2003). *The foundations of social research. Meaning and perspective in the research process.* London/Thousand Oaks, CA/New Delhi: SAGE.

Dahl, B. (2015). *Queer challenges in maternity care. A qualitative study about lesbian couples' experiences.* (PhD), University of Bergen. http://bora.uib. no/handle/1956/9621 (30.11.2016).

Dahl, B., Fylkesnes, A. M., Sorlie, V., & Malterud, K. (2013). Lesbian women's experiences with healthcare providers in the birthing context: A meta-ethnography. *Midwifery, 29*(6), 674–681. doi:10.1016/j.midw.2012.06.008

Dam, K., & Hall, E. O. (2016). Navigating in an unpredictable daily life: A metasynthesis on children's experiences living with a parent with severe mental illness. *Scand J Caring Sci, 30*(3), 442–457. doi:10.1111/scs.12285

Dickens, G. L., Lamont, E., & Gray, S. (2016). Mental health nurses' attitudes, behaviour, experience and knowledge regarding adults with a diagnosis of borderline personality disorder: Systematic, integrative literature review. *J Clin Nurs, 25*(13–14), 1848–1875. doi:10.1111/jocn.13202

Dixon-Woods, M., Agarwal, S., Jones, D., Young, B., & Sutton, A. (2005). Synthesising qualitative and quantitative evidence: A review of possible methods. *J Health Serv Res Policy, 10*(1), 45–53.:doi:10.1177/135581960501000110

Dixon-Woods, M., Booth, A., & Sutton, A. J. (2007). Synthesizing qualitative research: A review of published reports. *Qual Res, 7*, 375–422. doi:10.1177/ 1468794107078517

Dixon-Woods, M., Cavers, D., Agarwal, S., Annandale, E., Arthur, A., Harvey, J., et al. (2006). Conducting a critical interpretive synthesis of the literature on access to healthcare by vulnerable groups. *BMC Med Res Methodol, 6*, 35. doi:10.1186/1471-2288-6-35

Dobrow, M. J., Goel, V., & Upshur, R. E. (2004). Evidence-based health policy: Context and utilisation. *Soc Sci Med, 58*(1), 207–217. doi:10.1016/ S0277-9536(03)00166-7

Eakin, J. M., & Mykhalovskiy, E. (2003). Reframing the evaluation of qualitative health research: Reflections on a review of appraisal guidelines in the health sciences. *J Eval Clin Pract, 9*(2), 187–194.

Editorial Lancet. (1980). Aspirin after myocardial infarction. *The Lancet, 315*(8179), 1172–1173. doi:10.1016/S0140-6736(80)91626-8

Egger, M., Juni, P., Bartlett, C., Holenstein, F., & Sterne, J. (2003). How important are comprehensive literature searches and the assessment of trial quality in systematic reviews? Empirical study. *Health Technol. Assess., 7*(1), 1–76.

Fernee, C. R., Gabrielsen, L. E., Andersen, A. J. W., & Mesel, T. (2016). Unpacking the black box of wilderness therapy: A realist synthesis. *Qual Health Res.* doi:10.1177/1049732316655776

Finfgeld-Connett, D. (2018). *A guide to qualitative meta-synthesis.* New York and London: Routledge.

Finlay, L. (2008). Introducing reflexivity. In L. Finlay & B. Gough (Eds.), *Reflexivity A practical guide for researchers in health and social sciences* (pp. 1–49). Oxford: Wiley.

Fisher, M., Qureshi, H., Hardyman, W., & Homewood, J. (2006). *Using qualitative research in systematic reviews: Older people's views of hospital discharge.* http://www.Scie.Org.Uk/publications/reports/report09.Pdf (08.11.2016).

Fosse, A., Schaufel, M. A., Ruths, S., & Malterud, K. (2014). End-of-life expectations and experiences among nursing home patients and their relatives – A synthesis of qualitative studies. *Patient Educ Couns, 97*(1), 3–9. doi:10.1016/j.pec.2014.05.025

Foucault, M. (1988). Technologies of the self. In H. Gutman, M. Foucault, L. H. Martin, & P. H. Hutton (Eds.), *Technologies of the self: A seminar with Michel Foucault* (pp. 16–63). London: Tavistock.

France, E. F., Ring, N., Thomas, R., Noyes, J., Maxwell, M., & Jepson, R. (2014). A methodological systematic review of what's wrong with meta-ethnography reporting. *BMC Med Res Methodol, 14*(1), 1–16. doi:10.1186/1471-2288-14-119.

Frank, A. W. (2012). Practicing dialogical narrative analysis. In J. A. Holstein & J. F. Gubrium (Eds.), *Varieties of narrative analysis* (pp. 33–52). Los Angeles, CA: SAGE.

Frodeman, R. (2014). *Sustainable knowledge: A theory of interdisciplinarity.* Basingstoke: Macmillan.

Garfinkel, H. (1967). *Studies in ethnomethodology.* Englewood Cliffs, NJ: Prentice-Hall.

Geertz, C. (2000). *The interpretation of cultures: Selected essays.* New York: Basic Books.

Glaser, B., & Strauss, A. (1967). *The discovery of Grounded Theory: Strategies for qualitative research.* London: Wiedenfeld & Nicholson.

Glasziou, P., Meats, E., Heneghan, C., & Shepperd, S. (2008). What is missing from descriptions of treatment in trials and reviews? *Br Med J, 336*(7659), 1472–1474. doi:10.1136/bmj.39590.732037.47

Glenton, C., Colvin, C. J., Carlsen, B., Swartz, A., Lewin, S., Noyes, J., et al. (2013). Barriers and facilitators to the implementation of lay health worker programmes to improve access to maternal and child health: Qualitative evidence synthesis. *Cochrane Database Syst Rev, 10*, Cd010414. doi:10.1002/14651858.CD010414.pub2

Glenton, C., Lewin, S., & Gülmezoglu, A. M. (2016a). Expanding the evidence base for global recommendations on health systems: Strengths and challenges of the OptimizeMNH guidance process. *Implement Sci, 11*(1), 98. doi:10.1186/s13012-016-0470-y

Glenton, C., Lewin, S., & Norris, S. L. (2016b). Using evidence from qualitative research to develop who guidelines (Chapter 15). *Handbook for guideline development (2nd ed.).* Geneva: WHO.

Glover, J., Izzo, D., Odato, K., & Wang, L. (2006). EBM pyramid and EBM page generator. http://guides.Lib.Uci.Edu/ebm/pyramid (27.02.2017).

Gough, D., Oliver, S., & Thomas, J. (2017a). Introducing systematic reviews. In D. Gough, S. Oliver, & J. Thomas (Eds.), *An introduction to systematic reviews.* (2nd ed..pp. 1–17). London: SAGE.

Gough, D., Oliver, S., & Thomas, J. (Eds.). (2017b). *An introduction to systematic reviews. (2nd ed.)* London: SAGE.

Gough, D., & Thomas, J. (2017). Commonality and diversity in reviews. In D. Gough, S. Oliver, & J. Thomas (Eds.), *An introduction to systematic reviews. (2nd ed.,*(pp. 43–70). London: SAGE.

Government of Canada. Panel on research ethics. TCPS 2 (2014)—The latest edition of tri-council policy statement: Ethical conduct for research involving humans. http://www.Pre.Ethics.Gc.Ca/eng/policy-politique/initiatives/tcps2-eptc2/default/ (06.10.2018).

Grant, M. J. (2004). How does your searching grow? A survey of search preferences and the use of optimal search strategies in the identification of qualitative research. *Health Inform Libraries J, 21*(1), 21–32. doi:10.1111/j.1471-1842.2004.00483.x

Greenhalgh, T. (2012). Why do we always end up here? Evidence-based medicine's conceptual cul-de-sacs and some off-road alternative routes. *J Prim Health Care, 4*(2), 92–97.

Greenhalgh, T., Howick, J., & Maskrey, N. (2014). Evidence based medicine: A movement in crisis? *BMJ, 348*, g3725. doi:10.1136/bmj.g3725

Guyatt, G., Oxman, A. D., Akl, E. A., Kunz, R., Vist, G., Brozek, J., et al. (2011). GRADE guidelines: 1. Introduction—grade evidence profiles and summary of findings tables. *J Clin Epidemiol, 64*(4), 383–394. doi:10.1016/j.jclinepi.2010.04.026

Guyatt, G., Oxman, A. D., Vist, G. E., Kunz, R., Falck-Ytter, Y., Alonso-Coello, P., et al. (2008). GRADE: An emerging consensus on rating quality of evidence and strength of recommendations. *BMJ, 336*(7650), 924–926. doi:10.1136/bmj.39489.470347.AD

Hamberg, K., Johansson, E., Lindgren, G., & Westman, G. (1994). Scientific rigour in qualitative research – Examples from a study of women's health in family practice. *Fam Pract, 11*(2), 176–181.

Hannes, K., Booth, A., Harris, J., & Noyes, J. (2013). Celebrating methodological challenges and changes: Reflecting on the emergence and importance of the role of qualitative evidence in Cochrane reviews. *Systematic Reviews, 2*(1), 84. doi:10.1186/2046-4053-2-84

Hannes, K., & Macaitis, K. (2012). A move to more transparent and systematic approaches of qualitative evidence synthesis: Update of a review on published papers. *Qual Res, 12*(4), 402–442. doi:10.1177/1468794111432992

Haraway, D. (1991). Situated knowledges; the science question in feminism and the privilege of partial perspective. In D. Haraway (Ed.), *Simians, cyborgs, and women. The reinvention of nature* (pp. 183–201). New York: Routledge.

Higgins, J. P., & Green, S. (2011). Cochrane handbook for systematic reviews of interventions version 5.1.0 [updated March 2011]. http://handbook.cochrane.org/ (21.03.2017)

Hopewell, S., Loudon, K., Clarke, M. J., Oxman, A. D., & Dickersin, K. (2009). Publication bias in clinical trials due to statistical significance or direction of trial results. *Cochrane Database Syst Rev* (1). doi:10.1002/14651858. MR000006.pub3

Ioannidis, J. P. (2016). The mass production of redundant, misleading, and conflicted systematic reviews and meta-analyses. *Milbank Q, 94*(3), 485–514. doi:10.1111/1468-0009.12210

Jamtvedt, G. (2013). Systematiske oversikter om effekt av tiltak. *Norsk Epidemiologi, 23*(2), 119–124.

Jansen, K., Ruths, S., Malterud, K., & Schaufel, M. A. (2016). The impact of existential vulnerability for nursing home doctors in end-of-life care: A focus group study. *Patient Educ Couns, 99*(12): 2043–2048. Epub 16 Jul 12. doi: 10.1016/j.pec.2016.07.016.

Johansen, M. L., & Risor, M. B. (2016). What is the problem with medically unexplained symptoms for GPs? A meta-synthesis of qualitative studies. *Patient Educ Couns* doi:10.1016/j.pec.2016.11.015

Josselson, R. (2011). Narrative research. Constructing, deconstructing, and reconstructing story. In F. J. Wertz (Ed.), *Five ways of doing qualitative analysis. Phenomenological psychology, grounded theory, discourse analysis, narrative research, and intuitive inquiry* (pp. 224–242). New York: Guilford Press.

Kastner, M., Antony, J., Soobiah, C., Straus, S. E., & Tricco, A. C. (2016). Conceptual recommendations for selecting the most appropriate knowledge synthesis method to answer research questions related to complex evidence. *J Clin Epidemiol., 73*, 43–49. doi:10.1016/j.jclinepi.2015.11.022

Kastner, M., Tricco, A. C., Soobiah, C., Lillie, E., Perrier, L., Horsley, T., et al. (2012). What is the most appropriate knowledge synthesis method to conduct a review? Protocol for a scoping review. *BMC Med Res Methodol, 12*. doi:10.1186/1471-2288-12-114

Kelly, M. P., Heath, I., Howick, J., & Greenhalgh, T. (2015). The importance of values in evidence-based medicine. *BMC Med Ethics, 16*(1), 1–8. doi:10.1186/s12910-015-0063-3

Kuhn, T. S. (1962). *The structure of scientific revolutions.* Chicago, IL: University of Chicago Press.

Kuzel, A. (1999). Sampling in qualitative inquiry. In W. Miller & B. Crabtree (Eds.), *Doing qualitative research* (2nd ed., pp. 33–45). Thousand Oaks, CA: SAGE.

Kvale, S. (1996). *Interviews. An introduction to qualitative research interviewing.* Thousand Oaks, CA: SAGE.

Laliberte Rudman, D., Egan, M. Y., McGrath, C. E., Kessler, D., Gardner, P., King, J., et al. (2016). Low vision rehabilitation, age-related vision loss, and risk: A critical interpretive synthesis. *Gerontologist, 56*(3), e32–45. doi:10.1093/geront/gnv685

Lambert, H. C., McColl, M. A., Gilbert, J., Wong, J., Murray, G., & Shortt, S. E. (2005). Factors affecting long-term-care residents' decision-making processes as they formulate advance directives. *Gerontologist, 45*(5), 626–633.

Larun, L. (2011). *Kronisk utmattelsessyndrom. Kunnskap, aktivitet og utfordringer.* [Chronic Fatigue Syndrome. Knowledge, activity and challenges] (PhD). University of Bergen. (in Norwegian, English summary). http://bora.uib.no/handle/1956/5105 (14.03.2017)

Larun, L., & Malterud, K. (2007). Identity and coping experiences in chronic fatigue syndrome: A synthesis of qualitative studies. *Patient Educ Couns, 69*(1–3), 20–28.

Latour, B., & Woolgar, S. (1986). *Laboratory life: The construction of scientific facts* (New ed.). Princeton, NJ: Princeton University Press.

Lavis, J., Davies, H., Oxman, A., Denis, J. L., Golden-Biddle, K., & Ferlie, E. (2005). Towards systematic reviews that inform health care management and policy-making. *J Health Serv Res Policy, 10 (Suppl 1)*, 35–48. doi:10.1258/1355819054308549

Levin, A. (2001). The Cochrane Collaboration. *Ann Intern Med, 135*(4), 309–312. doi:10.7326/0003-4819-135-4-200108210-00035

Levitt, H. M., Bamberg, M., Creswell, J. W., Frost, D. M., Josselson, R., & Suarez-Orozco, C. (2018). Journal article reporting standards for qualitative primary, qualitative meta-analytic, and mixed methods research in psychology: The APA publications and communications board task force report. *Am Psychol, 73*(1), 26–46. doi:10.1037/amp0000151

Lewin, S., Booth, A., Glenton, C., Munthe-Kaas, H., Rashidian, A., Wainwright, M., et al. (2018). Applying grade-cerqual to qualitative evidence synthesis findings: Introduction to the series. *Implement Sci: IS, 13*(Suppl 1), 2. doi:10.1186/s13012-017-0688-3

Lewin, S., Bosch-Capblanch, X., Oliver, S., Akl, E. A., Vist, G. E., Lavis, J. N., et al. (2012). Guidance for evidence-informed policies about health systems: Assessing how much confidence to place in the research evidence. *PLoS Med, 9*(3), e1001187. doi:10.1371/journal.pmed.1001187

Lewin, S., Glenton, C., Munthe-Kaas, H., Carlsen, B., Colvin, C. J., Gülmezoglu, M., et al. (2015). Using qualitative evidence in decision making for health and social interventions: An approach to assess confidence in findings from qualitative evidence syntheses (GRADE-CERQual). *PLoS Med, 12*(10), e1001895. doi:10.1371/journal.pmed.1001895

Liberati, A., Altman, D. G., Tetzlaff, J., Mulrow, C., Gotzsche, P. C., Ioannidis, J. P., et al. (2009). The PRISMA statement for reporting systematic reviews and meta-analyses of studies that evaluate health care interventions: Explanation and elaboration. *J Clin Epidemiol, 62*(10), e1–34. doi: 10.1016/j.jclinepi.2009.06.006

Lock, A., & Strong, T. (2010). *Social constructionism: Sources and stirrings in theory and practice*. Cambridge: Cambridge University Press

Loder, E., Groves, T., Schroter, S., Merino, J. G., & Weber, W. (2016). Qualitative research and the BMJ. *BMJ, 352*. doi:10.1136/bmj.i641

Maanen, J. v. (2011). *Tales of the field. On writing ethnography*. Chicago, IL: University of Chicago Press.

MacLure, M. (2005). 'Clarity bordering on stupidity': Where's the quality in systematic review? *J Educ Policy, 20*(4), 393–416. doi:10.1080/02680930500131801

Major, C. H., & Savin-Baden, M. (2010). *An introduction to qualitative research synthesis. Managing the information explosion in social science research*. London/New York: Routledge.

Malinowski, B. (1944). *A scientific theory of culture*. Chapel Hill,: The University of North Carolina Press.

Malpass, A., Shaw, A., Sharp, D., Walter, F., Feder, G., Ridd, M., et al. (2009). "Medication career" or "moral career"? The two sides of managing antidepressants: A meta-ethnography of patients' experience of antidepressants. *Soc Sci Med, 68*(1), 154–168. doi:10.1016/j.socscimed.2008.09.068

Malterud, K. (1993). Shared understanding of the qualitative research process. Guidelines for the medical researcher. *FamPract, 10*(2), 201–206.

Malterud, K. (1995). The legitimacy of clinical knowledge: Towards a medical epistemology embracing the art of medicine. *Theor Med, 16*(2), 183–198.

Malterud, K. (2001a). The art and science of clinical knowledge: Evidence beyond measures and numbers. *Lancet, 358*(9279), 397–400. doi:10.1016/S0140-6736(01)05548-9

Malterud, K. (2001b). Qualitative research: Standards, challenges, and guidelines. *Lancet, 358*(9280), 483–488. doi:10.1016/S0140-6736(01)05627-6

Malterud, K. (2002). Reflexivity and metapositions: Strategies for appraisal of clinical evidence. *J Eval Clin Pract, 8*(2), 121–126.

Malterud, K. (2012). Systematic text condensation: A strategy for qualitative analysis. *Scand J Publ Health, 40*(8), 795–805. doi:10.1177/1403494812465030

Malterud, K. (2016). Theory and interpretation in qualitative studies from general practice: Why and how? *Scand. J Publ Health, 44*, 120–129. Epub December 128, 2015. doi:10.1177/1403494815621181

Malterud, K. (2017a). *Kvalitativ metasyntese som forskningsmetode i medisin og helsefag [Qualitative metasynthesis as a research method for medicine and health sciences] (in Norwegian).* Oslo: Universitetsforlaget.

Malterud, K. (2017b). *Kvalitative forskningsmetoder for medisin og helsefag. (4. utg.) [Qualitative research methods for medicine and health sciences] (in Norwegian, 4th ed.).* Oslo: Universitetsforlaget.

Malterud, K. (2019). The impact of evidence-based medicine on qualitative metasynthesis: Benefits to be harvested and warnings to be given. *Qual Health Res, 21*(1), 7–17. Epub 2018/2008/2031. doi.10.1177/1049732318795864

Malterud, K., Bjelland, A. K., & Elvbakken, K. T. (2016a). Evidence-based medicine – An appropriate tool for evidence-based health policy? A case study from Norway. *Health Res Policy Syst, 14*(1). doi:10.1186/s12961-016-0088-1

Malterud, K., Guassora, A. D., Reventlow, S., & Jutel, A. (2017). Embracing uncertainty to advance diagnosis in general practice. *B. J Gen Pract, 67*(659), 244–245. doi:10.3399/bjgp17X690941

Malterud, K., Siersma, V. D., & Guassora, A. D. (2016b). Sample size in qualitative interview studies: Guided by information power. *Qual Health Res, 26*(13), 1753–1760. Epub Nov 1727, 2015. doi::10.1177/1049732315617444

Malterud, K., & Ulriksen, K. (2010). Obesity in general practice: A focus group study on patient experiences. *Scand J Prim Health Care, 28*(4), 205–210. doi:10.3109/02813432.2010.526773

Malterud, K., & Ulriksen, K. (2011). Obesity, stigma, and responsibility in health care: A synthesis of qualitative studies. *Int J Qual Stud Health Well-being, 6*(4), 8404. doi:10.3402/qhw.v6i4.8404

Mays, N., Pope, C., & Popay, J. (2005). Systematically reviewing qualitative and quantitative evidence to inform management and policy-making in the health field. *J Health Serv Res Policy, 10(Suppl 1)*, 6–20.

McWhinney, I. R. (1989). "An acquaintance with particulars...". *Fam Med, 21*, 296–298.

Merriam Webster Dictionary. Metaphor. www.Merriam-webster.com/dictionary/metaphor (08.10.2018).

Merriam Webster Dictionary. Sustainable. www.Merriam-webster.Com/dictionary/sustainable (08.10.2018).

Merriam Webster Dictionary. Upcycle. www.Merriam-webster.Com/dictionary/upcycle (08.10.2018).

Migiro, S. O., & Magangi, B. A. (2011). Mixed methods: A review of literature and the future of the new research paradigm. *African J Business Manag. 5*(10), 3757–3764.

Miles, M. B., Huberman, A. M., & Saldaña, J. (2014). *Qualitative data analysis: A methods sourcebook* (3rd ed.). Los Angeles, CA: SAGE.

Moher, D., Glasziou, P., Chalmers, I., Nasser, M., Bossuyt, P. M., Korevaar, D. A., et al. (2016). Increasing value and reducing waste in biomedical research: Who's listening? *Lancet, 387*(10027), 1573–1586. doi:10.1016/S0140-6736(15)00307-4

Montgomery, K. (2006). *How doctors think: Clinical judgement and the practice of medicine.* Oxford: Oxford University Press.

Moreira, T. (2007). Entangled evidence: Knowledge making in systematic reviews in healthcare. *Sociol Health Illn, 29*(2), 180–197. doi:10.1111/j.1467-9566.2007.00531.x

Morrow, K. J., Gustavson, A. M., & Jones, J. (2016). Speaking up behaviours (safety voices) of healthcare workers: A metasynthesis of qualitative research studies. *Int J. Nurs Stud, 64*, 42–51. doi:10.1016/j.ijnurstu.2016.09.014

Morse, J. M. (1994). Going in "blind". *Qual Health Res, 4*, 3–5.

Munthe-Kaas, H. M., Hammerstrøm, K. T., Kurtze, N., & Nordlund, K. R. (2013). *Effects and experiences of interventions to promote continuity in residential child care institutions report from the Norwegian Knowledge Centre for the Health Services no. 4–2013.* www.Fhi.No/en/publ/2013/effects-and-experiences-of-interventions-to-promote-continuity-in-residenti/ (08.10.2018).

Murray, C., Turpin, M., Edwards, I., & Jones, M. (2015). A qualitative metasynthesis about challenges experienced in occupational therapy practice. *Br J Occup Ther, 78*(9), 534–546. doi:10.1177/0308022615586786

Mørland, B. (2014). *Kunnskapssenteret ti år [the Knowledge Centre Ten Years] (in Norwegian)* (Vol. 11). Oslo: Nasjonalt kunnskapssenter for helsetjen esten [The Norwegian Knowledge Centre for the Health Services]. www.dnms.no/index.php?setPublikasjon=true&seks_id=170263 (13.01.2015).

Nasjonalt kunnskapssenter for helsetjenesten. (2015). *Slik oppsummerer vi forskning [How to undertake systematic reviews] (in Norwegian)* www. Kunnskapssenteret.No/verktoy/slik-oppsummerer-vi-forskning (13.05.2015).

National Institute for Health Research. Governance, approvals and registration. www.Nihr.Ac.Uk/funding-and-support/funding-for-research-studies/manage-my-study/governance-approvals-and-registration.Htm (06.10.2018).

Noblit, G. W., & Hare, R. D. (1988). *Meta-ethnography: Synthesizing qualitative studies.* Newbury Park, CA: SAGE.

Noyes, J., Hannes, K., Booth, A., Harris, J., Harden, A., Popay, J., et al. (2015). Chapter 20: Qualitative research and Cochrane reviews. In: J. P. T. Higgins & S. Green S. (Eds.), *Cochrane Handbook for Systematic Reviews of Interventions*. Version 5.3.0 (updated October 2015). The Cochrane Collaboration. Http://handbook.Cochrane.Org/chapter_20/20_qualitative_research_and_cochrane_reviews.Htm (19.12.2016).

Noyes, J., & Lewin, S. (2011). Chapter 6: Supplemental guidance on selecting a method of qualitative evidence synthesis, and integrating qualitative evidence with Cochrane intervention reviews. In: J. Noyes, A. Booth, K. Hannes, A. Harden, J. Harris, S. Lewin & C. Lockwood. (Eds.), *Supplementary Guidance for Inclusion of Qualitative Research in Cochrane Systematic Reviews of Interventions*. The Cochrane Collaboration Qualitative Methods Group, 2011. http://methods.Cochrane.Org/qi/supplemental-handbook-guidance (21.03.2017).

O'Rourke, H. M., Duggleby, W., Fraser, K. D., & Jerke, L. (2015). Factors that affect quality of life from the perspective of people with dementia: A meta-synthesis. *J Am Geriatr Soc, 63*(1), 24–38. doi:10.1111/jgs.13178

O'Rourke, K. (2007). An historical perspective on meta-analysis: Dealing quantitatively with varying study results. *J R Soc Med, 100*(12), 579–582. doi:10.1258/jrsm.100.12.579

Oakley, A. (2017). Foreword. In D. Gough, S. Oliver, & J. Thomas (Eds.), *An introduction to systematic reviews*. (*2nd ed.,* pp. xiii–xvi). London: SAGE.

Oliver, S., Dickson, K., & Newman, M. (2012). Getting started with a review. In D. Gough, S. Oliver, & J. Thomas (Eds.), *An introduction to systematic reviews* (pp. 66–82). London: SAGE.

Orton, L., Lloyd-Williams, F., Taylor-Robinson, D., O'Flaherty, M., & Capewell, S. (2011). The use of research evidence in public health decision making processes: Systematic review. *PLoS One, 6*(7), e21704. doi::10.1371/journal.pone.0021704

Östlund, U., Kidd, L., Wengström, Y., & Rowa-Dewar, N. (2011). Combining qualitative and quantitative research within mixed method research designs: A methodological review. *Int J Nurs Stud*, 48(3), 369–383.

Oxford English Dictionary. Evidence. https://en.Oxforddictionaries.Com/definition/evidence (08.10.2018).

Oxman, A., & Guyatt, G. H. (1993). The science of reviewing research. *Ann N Y Acad Sci, 703*, 125–133; discussion 133–124.

Oxman, A., Lavis, J., Lewin, S., & Fretheim, A. (2010/2014). *Support tools for evidence-informed health policymaking (stp). Rapport fra Kunnskapssenteret nr. 04–2010.* http://www.Kunnskapssenteret.No/en/publications/support-tools-for-evidence-informed-health-policymaking-stp 16.09.2015).

Paterson, B. L., Thorne, S. E., Canam, C., & Jillings, C. (2001). Meta-method. In B. L. Paterson, S. E. Thorne, C. Canam, & C. Jillings (Eds.), *Meta-study of qualitative health research* (pp. 70–91). Thousand Oaks, CA: SAGE.

Patton, M. Q. (2015). *Qualitative research & evaluation methods: Integrating theory and practice* (4th ed.). Thousand Oaks, CA: SAGE.

Pawson, R., Greenhalgh, T., Harvey, G., & Walshe, K. (2005). Realist review – A new method of systematic review designed for complex policy interventions. *J Health Serv Res Policy, 10 Suppl 1*, 21–34. doi:10.1258/1355819054308530

Peterson, M. C., Holbrook, J. H., Von Hales, D., Smith, N. L., & Staker, L. V. (1992). Contributions of the history, physical examination, and laboratory investigation in making medical diagnoses. *West J Med, 156*(2), 163–165.

Petticrew, M. (2015). Time to rethink the systematic review catechism? Moving from 'what works' to 'what happens'. *Syst Rev, 4*, 36. doi:10.1186/s13643-015-0027-1

Plummer, K. (2003). *Intimate citizenship: Private decisions and public dialogues.* Seattle, WA: University of Washington Press.

Popay, J., Rogers, A., & Williams, G. (1998). Rationale and standards for the systematic review of qualitative literature in health services research. *Qual Health Res, 8*(3), 341–351. doi:10.1177/104973239800800305

Riese, H., Carlsen, B., & Glenton, C. (2014). Qualitative research synthesis: How the whole can be greater than the sum of its parts *Anthropol Action, 21*(2), 23–30.

Riessman, C. K. (2008). *Narrative methods for the human sciences.* Los Angeles, CA: SAGE.

Rivas, C., Matheson, L., Nayoan, J., Glaser, A., Gavin, A., Wright, P., et al. (2016). Ethnicity and the prostate cancer experience: A qualitative meta-synthesis. *Psycho-Oncology, 25*(10), 1147–1156. doi:10.1002/pon.4222

Rogge, M. M., Greenwald, M., & Golden, A. (2004). Obesity, stigma, and civilized oppression. *ANS Adv Nurs Sci, 27*(4), 301–315.

Rosvold, K. A. (2012). Gjenbruk. Store norske leksikon. Epub 29.01.2012. https://snl.No/gjenbruk (02.03.2017).

Sackett, D. L., Rosenberg, W. M., Gray, J. A., Haynes, R. B., & Richardson, W. S. (1996). Evidence based medicine: What it is and what it isn't. *BMJ, 312*(7023), 71–72. doi:10.1136/bmj.312.7023.71

Sackett, D. L., & Wennberg, J. E. (1997). Choosing the best research design for each question. *BMJ, 315*(7123), 1636.

Saini, M., & Shlonsky, A. (2012). *Systematic synthesis of qualitative research.* Oxford: Oxford University Press.

Sandelowski, M. (2012). Metasynthesis of qualitative research. In H. Cooper, P. M. Camic, D. L. Long, A. T. Panter, D. Rindskopf, & K. J. Sher (Eds.), *APA Handbook of research methods in psychology, vol 2: Research designs: Quantitative, qualitative, neuropsychological, and biological* (pp. 19–36). Washington, DC: American Psychological Association.

Sandelowski, M., & Barroso, J. (2007). *Handbook of synthesizing qualitative research.* New York: Springer Publishing.

Santiago-Delefosse, M., Gavin, A., Bruchez, C., Roux, P., & Stephen, S. L. (2016). Quality of qualitative research in the health sciences: Analysis of the common criteria present in 58 assessment guidelines by expert users. *Soc Sci Med, 148*, 142–151. doi:10.1016/j.socscimed.2015.11.007

Schünemann, H. J., Fretheim, A., & Oxman, A. D. (2006). Improving the use of research evidence in guideline development: 13. Applicability, transferability and adaptation. *Health Res Policy Systems, 4*(1), 25. doi:10.1186/1478-4505-4-25

Schutz, A. (1962). *Collected papers.* Nijhoff: The Hague.

Shaneyfelt, T. (2016). Pyramids are guides not rules: The evolution of the evidence pyramid. *Evid Based Med, 21*(4), 121–122. doi:10.1136/ebmed-2016-110498

Shaw, R. (2015). Broadening the evidence base and the mind when thinking about mixed methods research. *Evid Based Med, 20*(2), 80. doi:10.1136/ebmed-2014-110165

Sibeoni, J., Orri, M., Colin, S., Valentin, M., Pradère, J., & Revah-Levy, A. (2017). The lived experience of anorexia nervosa in adolescence, comparison of the points of view of adolescents, parents, and professionals: A meta-synthesis. *Int J Nurs Stud, 65*, 25–34. doi:10.1016/j.ijnurstu.2016.10.006

Smith, L. K., Pope, C., & Botha, J. L. (2005). Patients' help-seeking experiences and delay in cancer presentation: A qualitative synthesis. *Lancet, 366*(9488), 825–831.

Smith, R., & Rennie, D. (2014). Evidence-based medicine – An oral history. *JAMA, 311*(4), 365–367. doi:10.1001/jama.2013.286182

Snilstveit, B., Oliver, S., & Vojtkova, M. (2012). Narrative approaches to systematic review and synthesis of evidence for international development policy and practice. *J Developm Effectiveness, 4*(3), 409–429. doi:10.1080/19439342.2012.710641

Sollaci, L. B., & Pereira, M. G. (2004). The introduction, methods, results, and discussion (IMRAD) structure: A fifty-year survey. *J Med Libr Assoc, 92*(3), 364–367.

Spiegelhalter, D. J., Myles, J. P., Jones, D. R., & Abrams, K. R. (2000). Bayesian methods in health technology assessment: A review. *Health Technol Assess, 4*(38), 1–130.

Statistics Norway. (2013). *Statistisk årbok.* Oslo.

Steihaug, S., Johannessen, A.-K., Ådnanes, M., Paulsen, B., & Mannion, R. (2016). Challenges in achieving collaboration in clinical practice: The case of Norwegian health care. *Int J Integrated Care, 16*(3), 3. doi10.5334/ijic.2217.

Stern, P. N., & Harris, C. C. (1985). Women's health and the self-care paradox: A model to guide self-care readiness. *Health Care Women Int., 6*(1–3), 151–163. doi:10.1080/07399338509515689

Stige, B., Malterud, K., & Midtgarden, T. (2009). Toward an agenda for evaluation of qualitative research. *Qual Health Res, 19*(10), 1504–1516. doi:10.1177/1049732309348501

Tan, S. Y., & Melendez-Torres, G. J. (2016). A systematic review and meta-synthesis of barriers and facilitators to negotiating consistent condom use among sex workers in Asia. *Culture, health & sexuality, 18*(3), 249–264. doi:10.1080/13691058.2015.1077994

Teddlie, C., & Tashakkori, A. (2009). *Foundations of mixed methods research. Integrating quantitative and qualitative approaches in the social and behavioral sciences.* Thousand Oaks, CA: SAGE.

The Joanna Briggs Institute. (2015). *The Joanna Briggs Institute reviewers' manual 2015. Methodology for JBI scoping reviews.* http://joannabriggs.

Org/assets/docs/sumari/reviewers-manual_methodology-for-jbi-scoping-reviews_2015_v2.Pdf (21.03.2017).

Thomas, J., & Harden, A. (2008). Methods for the thematic synthesis of qualitative research in systematic reviews. *BMC Med Res Methodol., 8*, 45. doi:10.1186/1471-2288-8-45

Thorne, S. (2008). *Interpretive description*. Walnut Creek. CA: Left Coast Press, Inc.

Thorne, S. (2015). Qualitative metasynthesis: A technical exercise or a source of new knowledge? *Psycho-Oncology.* doi:10.1002/pon.3944

Thorne, S. (2017). Metasynthetic madness: What kind of monster have we created? *Qual Health Res, 27*(1), 3–12. doi:10.1177/1049732316679370

Thorne, S., Jensen, L., Kearney, M. H., Noblit, G., & Sandelowski, M. (2004). Qualitative metasynthesis: Reflections on methodological orientation and ideological agenda. *Qual Health Res, 14*(10), 1342–1365. doi:10.1177/1049732304269888

Tong, A., Flemming, K., McInnes, E., Oliver, S., & Craig, J. (2012). Enhancing transparency in reporting the synthesis of qualitative research: ENTREQ. *BMC Med Res Methodol, 12*, 181. doi:10.1186/1471-2288-12-181

Tong, A., Sainsbury, P., & Craig, J. (2007). Consolidated criteria for reporting qualitative research (COREQ): A 32-item checklist for interviews and focus groups. *Int J Qual Health Care, 19*. doi:10.1093/intqhc/mzm042

Toye, F., Seers, K., Allcock, N., Briggs, M., Carr, E., & Barker, K. (2014). Meta-ethnography 25 years on: Challenges and insights for synthesising a large number of qualitative studies. *BMC Med Res Methodol, 14*, 80. doi:10.1186/1471-2288-14-80

Tricco, A. C., Antony, J., Soobiah, C., Kastner, M., MacDonald, H., Cogo, E., et al. (2016). Knowledge synthesis methods for integrating qualitative and quantitative data: A scoping review reveals poor operationalization of the methodological steps. *J Clin Epidemiol, 73*, 29–35. doi:10.1016/j.jclinepi.2015.12.011

Turner, S. P. (1980). *Sociological explanation as translation*. New York: Cambridge University Press.

Vetlesen, A.-J. (1994). *Perception, empathy, and judgment: An inquiry into the preconditions of moral performance*. University Park: Pennsylvania State University Press.

Vohra, J. U., Brazil, K., & Szala-Meneok, K. (2006). The last word: Family members' descriptions of end-of-life care in long-term care facilities. *J Palliat Care, 22*(1), 33–39.

Voldbjerg, S. L., Gronkjaer, M., Sorensen, E. E., & Hall, E. O. (2016). Newly graduated nurses' use of knowledge sources: A meta-ethnography. *J Adv Nurs, 72*(8), 1751–1765. doi:10.1111/jan.12914

Walsh, D., & Downe, S. (2005). Meta-synthesis method for qualitative research: A literature review. *J Adv Nurs, 50*(2), 204–211. doi:10.1111/j.1365-2648.2005.03380.x

White, D. G. (2001). Evaluating evidence and making judgements of study quality: Loss of evidence and risks to policy and practice decisions. *Critical Public Health, 11*(1), 3–17. doi:10.1080/09581590010028228

Whiting, P. F., Rutjes, A. W., Westwood, M. E., Mallett, S., Deeks, J. J., Reitsma, J. B., et al. (2011). Quadas-2: A revised tool for the quality assessment of diagnostic accuracy studies. *Ann Intern Med, 155*(8), 529–536. doi:10.7326/0003-4819-155-8-201110180-00009

Wilson, H. S., & Hutchinson, S. A. (1996). Methodologic mistakes in Grounded Theory. *Nurs Res, 45*(2), 122–124.

Wong, G. (2016). Knowledge synthesis approaches –Spoilt for choice? *J Clin Epidemiol, 73*, 8–10. doi:10.1016/j.jclinepi.2015.08.031

Wong, G., Greenhalgh, T., Westhorp, G., Buckingham, J., & Pawson, R. (2013). Rameses publication standards: Realist syntheses. *BMC Med, 11.* doi:10.1186/1741-7015-11-21

World Health Organization. Task shifting: Global recommendations and guidelines. 2008. http://www.Who.Int/workforcealliance/knowledge/resources/taskshifting_guidelines/en/ (04.09.2018).

World Medical Association. (2013). WMA Declaration of Helsinki – Ethical principles for medical research involving human subjects. http://www.wma.net/en/30publications/10policies/b3/ (02.09.2014)

Yablonsky, A. M., Barbero, E. D., & Richardson, J. W. (2016). Hard is normal: Military families' transitions within the process of deployment. *Res Nurs Health 39*(1), 42–56. doi:10.1002/nur.21701

Index